Depression and Personality

Series Editors

Mariane Krause, Faculty of Social Sciences, Pontificia Universidad Católica de Chile, Santiago, Chile

Guillermo De La Parra, Department of Psychiatry, Pontificia Universidad Católica de Chile, Santiago, Chile

Alemka Tomicic, Faculty of Psychology, Universidad Diego Portales, Santiago, Chile

The Depression and Personality book series presents cutting edge knowledge regarding the causes, treatment, and prevention of depression from a perspective that takes into account the interaction between depression and personality and the influences of multiple dimensions that contribute to the development, maintenance, and exacerbation of depression in different populations. The series is published in collaboration with the Millennium Institute for Research in Depression and Personality (MIDAP), a scientific center of excellence in Chile made up of psychologists, psychiatrists and professionals from various areas of social sciences and health, who seek to generate knowledge based on a multidimensional understanding of depression.

MIDAP's characteristic multidimensional and multidisciplinary approach implies the development of an empirically-based model that takes into account the etiology, prevention, intervention, and rehabilitation of depression. This multidimensional and multidisciplinary model is evidenced in the titles of the series, which cover, individually or in combination, the following topics:

1. Basic bio-psycho-social structures and processes involved in depression and its interaction with the personality.
2. Health promotion and psychosocial intervention strategies that would prevent early conditions associated with the development of depression and personality dysfunction.
3. Psychotherapeutic interventions and mechanisms involved in symptomatic relief and change processes in diverse types of depressive patients.
4. Rehabilitation and reintegration interventions oriented to reduce the chronicity of depression and to maintain gains after treatment, as well as, topics regarding early-life maltreatment and co-morbid personality dysfunction as risk factors of chronic or recurrent courses of depression.

Álvaro Jiménez-Molina • Vania Martínez
Editors

New Perspectives on Suicidal Behavior

Cultural Context, Clinical Assessment, and Intervention

Springer

Editors
Álvaro Jiménez-Molina
Faculty of Psychology and Humanities
Universidad San Sebastián
Santiago, RM - Santiago, Chile

Vania Martínez
Faculty of Medicine
Universidad de Chile
Santiago, RM - Santiago, Chile

ISSN 2662-3587 ISSN 2662-3595 (electronic)
Depression and Personality
ISBN 978-3-031-96036-9 ISBN 978-3-031-96037-6 (eBook)
https://doi.org/10.1007/978-3-031-96037-6

This Springer imprint is published by the registered company Springer Nature Switzerland AG
The registered company address is: Gewerbestrasse 11, 6330 Cham, Switzerland

Contents

Chapter 1
Introduction

Álvaro Jiménez-Molina and Vania Martínez

Suicide and suicidal behaviors pose a critical challenge to global public health, with more than 700,000 deaths annually, accounting for approximately 1.3% of all deaths (Knipe et al., 2022). Despite being a preventable cause, it is the fourth leading cause of death among young people aged 15–29. Globally, the prevalence of lifetime suicidal ideation is estimated at 9.2%, while suicide attempts reach 2.7% (Turecki & Brent, 2016). However, suicide rates vary significantly between countries (Knipe et al., 2022).

Research has shown that suicide risk results from the complex and dynamic interaction of biological, psychological, cultural, environmental, and social factors over time. Among the most prominent are certain personality traits, such as impulsivity, hopelessness, pessimism about the future, and feelings of defeat and entrapment (Turecki et al., 2019; Zortea et al., 2020). Adverse childhood experiences, particularly physical or sexual abuse, are also strongly linked to an increased risk of suicide in adulthood (Turecki et al., 2019). Additionally, a family history of suicide or exposure to suicidal behaviors significantly raises the likelihood of someone engaging in suicidal actions (Martínez et al., 2023). In recent years, greater attention

Á. Jiménez-Molina (✉)
Faculty of Psychology and Humanities, Universidad San Sebastián, Santiago, RM - Santiago, Chile

Millennium Institute for Research in Depression and Personality (MIDAP), Santiago, Chile

Nucleus to Improve the Mental Health of Adolescents and Youths (Imhay), Santiago, Chile
e-mail: alvaro.jimenez@uss.cl

V. Martínez
Millennium Institute for Research in Depression and Personality (MIDAP), Santiago, Chile

Nucleus to Improve the Mental Health of Adolescents and Youths (Imhay), Santiago, Chile

Faculty of Medicine, Universidad de Chile, Santiago, RM - Santiago, Chile

Mental Health Department, Ministerio de Salud, Santiago, Chile

Á. Jiménez-Molina, V. Martínez (eds.), *New Perspectives on Suicidal Behavior*, Depression and Personality, https://doi.org/10.1007/978-3-031-96037-6_1

has been given to social factors in studies on suicidal behavior, such as isolation, lack of social support, and socioeconomic disadvantages, including poverty and unemployment (Bantjes et al., 2016).

Despite advances in understanding the epidemiology and identifying risk factors associated with suicidal behavior (Knipe et al., 2022), reliable predictors that accurately determine who is at greatest risk remain elusive. Moreover, the interaction between these risk factors is not yet fully understood. Although the strongest predictor of suicide is a previous attempt, only about 10% of those who survive an attempt ultimately die by suicide (Knipe et al., 2022), and men are more likely to die on their first attempt (Bennett et al., 2023).

The presence of mental disorders significantly increases the risk of suicide, with studies showing that up to 90% of those who die by suicide had a diagnosable psychiatric disorder (Cavanagh et al., 2003). However, since most individuals with mental illnesses do not attempt or die by suicide, the presence of a mental disorder alone is not a sufficient risk marker. Similarly, while protective factors such as optimism, resilience, social connection, and support have been identified (Zortea et al., 2020), the mechanisms of recovery from suicidal thoughts and behaviors remain poorly understood.

Additionally, we still lack a comprehensive understanding of the factors contributing to the high suicide rates among Indigenous populations and the LGBTQ+ community. It is unclear whether known risk factors for suicide have the same impact in these communities, and there is a scarcity of data on specific protective factors in these groups.

The United Nations Sustainable Development Goals (SDGs) (United Nations, 2015) have highlighted suicide reduction as a key target for improving global health by 2030, identifying suicide mortality as an indicator of national well-being. While several governments have recognized the need to implement effective programs to prevent suicide and self-harm (Platt et al., 2019; WHO, 2021), evidence on the effectiveness of these interventions remains limited and contradictory (Lewitzka et al., 2019; Schlichthorst et al., 2023). Despite some therapeutic interventions showing effectiveness in reducing suicide risk (Turecki & Brent, 2016), significant knowledge gaps persist, underscoring the need to continue developing strategies at both public health and clinical levels. Although the universal, selective, and indicated (USI) prevention model has provided a helpful framework, more research is needed to determine which strategies are most effective and how different levels of intervention interact. Evidence is also limited on how to effectively implement suicide prevention and postvention programs in institutions such as hospitals, schools, and local governments (Andriessen et al., 2019; Platt et al., 2019).

In high-income countries, 80% of people who die by suicide had contact with primary care services in the year prior to their death, highlighting these encounters as critical intervention opportunities (Knipe et al., 2022; Walby et al., 2018). While studies have examined clinical management after hospitalization for suicidal behavior, more evidence is needed to identify best practices in the assessment, treatment, and follow-up of these patients. A meta-analysis spanning five decades of research reveals that the predictive ability of current systems is no better than chance

(Franklin et al., 2017). Similarly, a meta-analysis on the effectiveness of suicide prevention interventions suggests that their efficacy has not improved over the past five decades (Fox et al., 2020).

Significant advances have been made in understanding and preventing suicidal behavior over the past few decades, yet significant challenges persist. Traditionally, suicide prevention has been approached from a predominantly clinical perspective, focusing on interventions led by mental health professionals that address individual risk factors, such as family history, mental disorders, substance use, and stressful life events. While these perspectives are crucial, they must be complemented with strategies that consider the broader social context in which individuals live, incorporating social, economic, and cultural determinants of suicide (Pirkis et al., 2024; Sinyor et al., 2024).

One of the primary challenges in suicide research is the lack of studies conducted in regions with the greatest need. Even though 80% of suicides occur in low- and middle-income countries (LMICs), only 15% of suicide-related research originates from these areas (Knipe et al., 2022). Although high-income countries (HICs) have managed to reduce their suicide rates significantly, LMICs have not been able to achieve similar progress. This imbalance highlights the urgent need to generate more knowledge in LMICs and adapt prevention strategies to their specific cultural and socioeconomic realities.

Furthermore, the emerging field of critical suicidology has recently challenged the dominant narrative that most individuals who die by suicide experience mental disorders. It critiques conventional approaches for reinforcing a Western biomedical perspective in suicide prevention, which may not be fully applicable to other contexts (White et al., 2022). Addressing these challenges is essential to closing knowledge gaps and developing more culturally and contextually relevant suicide prevention and postvention strategies.

In response to these complexities, this book, part of the *Depression and Personality* book series, offers a valuable opportunity to reflect on insights gained in suicide research across diverse contexts. Featuring contributions from researchers from various countries and perspectives, it provides a comprehensive overview of current knowledge on suicide, including its theoretical frameworks, sociocultural dimensions, clinical assessment, and intervention strategies. As part of this comprehensive approach, experts emphasize using person-centered, non-stigmatizing language to foster a more respectful dialogue. For this reason, the following terms were discouraged in this book: *committing suicide* and *suicidal person*, among others (Mishara & Dargis, 2019; Public Health Agency of Canada, 2018).

The book is divided into two sections. The first section focuses on the complexities of suicidal behavior, examining key psychological models and cultural dimensions that influence it, including the experiences of transgender and Mapuche communities.

Chapter 2, "Theorizing Suicidal Behavior," offers an in-depth overview of the most relevant findings in the psychology of suicidal behavior, focusing on integrative theoretical models. Drawing on the distinction between first- and second-generation psychological theories of suicide, the chapter examines the current state of these models, exploring their implications for research and clinical practice while addressing the challenges they present. The chapter offers a critical perspective on the development of contemporary theoretical models in suicidology, underscoring the lack of significant progress, particularly in integrating sociocultural dimensions and gaining a deeper understanding of the mechanisms underlying suicidal behavior. Additionally, the chapter explores the potential contributions of critical suicidology approaches to advancing these models.

Chapter 3, "On the Psychodynamics of Suicidal Behaviors," shifts focus to the psychodynamics of suicidal behavior, with a particular emphasis on depressive personality traits. From a psychoanalytic viewpoint, the chapter examines how feelings of rejection, guilt, low self-esteem, and inward-directed anger contribute to suicidal ideation, identifying disconnection, hopelessness, and psychological pain as central factors in understanding these behaviors. The chapter also discusses impulsivity and "acting out" as coping mechanisms for emotional distress. It concludes by exploring how psychotherapy can effectively modify maladaptive self-representations and object relations, promoting psychological growth and providing therapeutic relief from destructive patterns.

Chapter 4, "Reexamining the Role of Suicidal Behavior in Personality Disorder: Current Diagnostic Considerations and Cultural Variability," delves into the intricate relationship between personality disorders and suicidal behavior. The chapter emphasizes the need to integrate frameworks such as the Dual-System Model and Suicide Crisis Syndrome into the Alternative Model for Personality Disorders (AMPD), offering insights into the mechanisms that perpetuate and develop suicidal behaviors. This chapter also contrasts modern diagnostic approaches such as the ICD-11 and AMPD with traditional frameworks such as the DSM-5, advocating for a dimensional approach. Cultural variability in the expression of personality disorders and their relationship to suicidality is also explored, underscoring the importance of culturally sensitive prevention and treatment strategies.

The last two chapters in the first section delve into the concepts of health, illness, and responses to suicide within Mapuche communities, as well as suicidal behaviors among transgender individuals, examining their implications for both research and clinical practice. These discussions reveal how gender-related factors and the social determinants of suicide, as identified in research, are shaped by specific cultural meanings, norms, and beliefs.

Chapter 5, "Resilience and Gender Affirmation: Coping Suicidality in Transgender and Gender Nonconforming People," centers on the elevated rates of suicidal behavior among transgender and gender non-conforming (TGNC) individuals who experience systemic discrimination and marginalization. The chapter explores the Minority Stress Model, which links societal stigma and oppression to higher rates of suicidality and psychopathology in TGNC populations. They also present a model that examines the development of gender identity and its connection to suicidal ideation in TGNC youth. Furthermore, the chapter highlights the protective role of gender affirmation processes in reducing suicidal behavior, emphasizing their importance in fostering well-being within TGNC communities, particularly in Latin America.

Chapter 6, "Understanding Suicidal Behavior in the Context of Mapuche Culture," shifts focus to the cultural and spiritual dimensions that influence the understanding of health, well-being, and suicidal behavior in Indigenous populations, with a specific emphasis on the Mapuche of southern Chile. Drawing on two *trawuns* (discussions) with Mapuche communities, the chapter explores their beliefs about health and illness, underscoring the crucial role of spirituality in shaping their perspectives on suicide. A clinical case is also analyzed from a transcultural standpoint, illustrating the conflict between Christian and Mapuche worldviews. The chapter emphasizes the need to collaborate with Indigenous spiritual guides to incorporate cultural meanings and practices into mental health treatments for Indigenous individuals at risk of suicide.

The book's second section focuses on evaluating and managing suicide risk, providing an overview of tools and strategies for early detection, assessment, and clinical intervention. It explores suicide prevention and postvention strategies across diverse settings, including clinical, educational, and community environments, emphasizing approaches that have proven effective in reducing suicidal ideation and attempts. Moreover, it highlights the increasing role of digital technologies in suicide prevention, particularly in expanding access to mental health care for adolescents and young people, as well as in resource-limited settings.

Chapter 7, "Comprehensive Understanding of Young People Suicide Risk Assessment and Intervention," explores the high incidence and persistence of suicidal ideation among young people. It examines risk and protective factors for youth suicide, the role of social determinants of health, and tools for screening and assessing suicide risk. Additionally, it discusses interventions across clinical, community, and digital settings, as well as the barriers—particularly stigma—that hinder timely access to mental health care.

Chapter 8, "The Role of Digital Technology in Youth Suicide Prevention," examines the role of digital interventions in preventing suicide and related behaviors. The chapter reviews the effectiveness of these interventions at various levels (USI), highlighting their benefits and limitations across different populations and settings, such as schools and mental health services. The chapter also addresses the methodological, technical, and ethical challenges in improving these interventions' acceptability, feasibility, safety, and effectiveness, offering strategies to enhance their real-world implementation and scalability.

Chapter 9, "Culturally Sensitive Suicide Prevention Programs: Addressing Indigenous Peoples in Latin America and the Caribbean," explores the cultural dimensions of suicide prevention in Indigenous communities. It starts by examining the beliefs, perceptions, and practices related to death and suicide in various Indigenous groups across Latin America and the Caribbean, assessing the impact of suicide on individuals, families, and communities. The chapter also maps out suicide prevention policies specifically tailored to these populations, providing recommendations for designing and implementing culturally sensitive and locally relevant interventions. The chapter concludes that the effectiveness of suicide prevention and postvention initiatives is enhanced when they incorporate elements that align with the worldview and cultural values of each Indigenous group.

The final two chapters of this section focus on the experiences of suicide loss survivors and postvention. These aspects have received less attention in suicide behavior research and prevention programs.

Chapter 10, "Suicide Bereavement and Postvention: What Do We Know and What Should We Know?" offers a comprehensive overview of the current knowledge and gaps in suicide bereavement and postvention, addressing the challenges faced in research, clinical practice, and program implementation across various settings (community, health services, and schools). The chapter explores suicide bereavement experiences and examines a range of survivor support strategies, including psychotherapy, community-based postvention, and suicide bereavement support groups. They conclude by emphasizing the critical importance of incorporating the experiences of suicide survivors as a key element in improving the understanding, prevention, and postvention of suicide.

Chapter 11, "The Impact of Suicide on Clinical Teams: Exploring the Needs of Mental Health Professionals," delves into the emotional and professional impact of a patient's suicide on healthcare professionals, particularly those in mental health. Drawing on a review of existing literature and an exploratory study of therapists who have lost patients to suicide, the chapter underscores the significant emotional toll on clinicians, which can manifest as sadness, anger, frustration, guilt, self-doubt, and questioning of their clinical abilities. The chapter not only examines the immediate and long-term effects of suicide on professionals' careers but also offers recommendations for supporting clinicians in coping with these traumatic experiences, emphasizing the importance of providing individual and group psychological support to clinical teams within healthcare institutions.

Overall, this book examines current challenges in suicide research, clinical practice, and prevention. By integrating theoretical insights with practical approaches, research findings, and actionable recommendations, the book underscores the importance of culturally sensitive and inclusive strategies for addressing global challenges in suicide prevention and postvention.

Acknowledgments This manuscript was supported by ANID—Millennium Science Initiative Program—AIM23_0002 and NCS2021_081, ANID—Fondecyt Project N° 1221230, and ANID—FONIS SA23I018.

References

Andriessen, K., Krysinska, K., Hill, N. T. M., Reifels, L., Robinson, J., Reavley, N., & Pirkis, J. (2019). Effectiveness of interventions for people bereaved through suicide: A systematic review of controlled studies of grief, psychosocial and suicide-related outcomes. *BMC Psychiatry, 19*(1), 49. https://doi.org/10.1186/s12888-019-2020-z

Bantjes, J., Iemmi, V., Coast, E., Channer, K., Leone, T., McDaid, D., Palfreyman, A., Stephens, B., & Lund, C. (2016). Poverty and suicide research in low- and middle-income countries: Systematic mapping of literature published in English and a proposed research agenda. *Global mental health (Cambridge, England), 3*, e32. https://doi.org/10.1017/gmh.2016.27

Bennett, S., Robb, K. A., Zortea, T. C., Dickson, A., Richardson, C., & O'Connor, R. C. (2023). Male suicide risk and recovery factors: A systematic review and qualitative metasynthesis of two decades of research. *Psychological Bulletin, 149*(7–8), 371–417. https://doi.org/10.1037/bul0000397

Cavanagh, J. T., Carson, A. J., Sharpe, M., & Lawrie, S. M. (2003). Psychological autopsy studies of suicide: A systematic review. *Psychological Medicine, 33*(3), 395–405. https://doi.org/10.1017/s0033291702006943

Fox, K. R., Huang, X., Guzmán, E. M., Funsch, K. M., Cha, C. B., Ribeiro, J. D., & Franklin, J. C. (2020). Interventions for suicide and self-injury: A meta-analysis of randomized controlled trials across nearly 50 years of research. *Psychological Bulletin, 146*(12), 1117–1145. https://doi.org/10.1037/bul0000305

Franklin, J. C., Ribeiro, J. D., Fox, K. R., Bentley, K. H., Kleiman, E. M., Huang, X., Musacchio, K. M., Jaroszewski, A. C., Chang, B. P., & Nock, M. K. (2017). Risk factors for suicidal thoughts and behaviors: A meta-analysis of 50 years of research. *Psychological Bulletin, 143*(2), 187–232. https://doi.org/10.1037/bul0000084

Knipe, D., Padmanathan, P., Newton-Howes, G., Chan, L. F., & Kapur, N. (2022). Suicide and self-harm. *Lancet (London, England), 399*(10338), 1903–1916. https://doi.org/10.1016/S0140-6736(22)00173-8

Lewitzka, U., Sauer, C., Bauer, M., & Felber, W. (2019). Are national suicide prevention programs effective? A comparison of 4 verum and 4 control countries over 30 years. *BMC Psychiatry, 19*(1), 158. https://doi.org/10.1186/s12888-019-2147-y

Martínez, V., Jiménez-Molina, Á., & Gerber, M. M. (2023). Social contagion, violence, and suicide among adolescents. *Current Opinion in Psychiatry, 36*(3), 237–242. https://doi.org/10.1097/YCO.0000000000000858

Mishara, B. L., & Dargis, L. (2019). Systematic comparison of recommendations for safe messaging about suicide in public communications. *Journal of Affective Disorders, 244*, 124–154. https://doi.org/10.1016/j.jad.2018.09.031

Pirkis, J., Dandona, R., Silverman, M., Khan, M., & Hawton, K. (2024). Preventing suicide: A public health approach to a global problem. *The Lancet. Public Health, 9*(10), e787–e795. https://doi.org/10.1016/S2468-2667(24)00149-X

Platt, S., Arensman, E., & Rezaeian, M. (2019). National suicide prevention strategies - Progress and challenges. *Crisis, 40*(2), 75–82. https://doi.org/10.1027/0227-5910/a000587

Public Health Agency of Canada, Centre for Suicide Prevention and l'Association québécoise de prévention du suicide. (2018). *Language Matters: Safe Communication for Suicide Prevention* https://www.canada.ca/en/public-health/services/publications/healthy-living/language-matters-safe-communication-suicide-prevention.html

Schlichthorst, M., Reifels, L., Spittal, M., Clapperton, A., Scurrah, K., Kolves, K., Platt, S., Pirkis, J., & Krysinska, K. (2023). Evaluating the effectiveness of components of national suicide prevention strategies. *Crisis, 44*(4), 318–328. https://doi.org/10.1027/0227-5910/a000887

Sinyor, M., Silverman, M., Pirkis, J., & Hawton, K. (2024). The effect of economic downturn, financial hardship, unemployment, and relevant government responses on suicide. *The Lancet. Public health, 9*(10), e802–e806. https://doi.org/10.1016/S2468-2667(24)00152-X

Turecki, G., & Brent, D. A. (2016). Suicide and suicidal behaviour. *Lancet (London, England), 387*(10024), 1227–1239. https://doi.org/10.1016/S0140-6736(15)00234-2

Turecki, G., Brent, D. A., Gunnell, D., O'Connor, R. C., Oquendo, M. A., Pirkis, J., & Stanley, B. H. (2019). Suicide and suicide risk. *Nature Reviews. Disease Primers, 5*(1), 74. https://doi.org/10.1038/s41572-019-0121-0

United Nations. (2015). *Transforming our world: The 2030 agenda for sustainable development* (A/RES/70/1). https://sustainabledevelopment.un.org/post2015/transformingourworld/publication

Walby, F. A., Myhre, M. Ø., & Kildahl, A. T. (2018). Contact with mental health services prior to suicide: A systematic review and meta-analysis. *Psychiatric Services (Washington, D.C.), 69*(7), 751–759. https://doi.org/10.1176/appi.ps.201700475

White, J., Marsh, I., Kral, M., & Morris, J. (2022). *Critical suicidology: Transforming suicide research and prevention for the 21st century*. University of Chicago Press.

World Health Organization. (2021). *LIVE LIFE: An implementation guide for suicide prevention in countries*. World Health Organization.

Zortea, T. C., Cleare, S., Melson, A. J., Wetherall, K., & O'Connor, R. C. (2020). Understanding and managing suicide risk. *British Medical Bulletin, 134*(1), 73–84. https://doi.org/10.1093/bmb/ldaa013

Part I
Suicidal Behavior in Context: Rethinking Psychological Models and Cultural Dimensions

Chapter 2
Theorizing Suicidal Behavior

Álvaro Jiménez-Molina

2.1 Why Is Our Knowledge About Suicidal Behaviors Still Insufficient?

Theoretical models in psychology are generally constructed to describe, explain, or predict empirical phenomena. These models provide criteria that guide the selection of variables and facilitate both the generation and testing of hypotheses, using various data types to understand or explain a specific phenomenon.

Over the past four decades, the development of various psychological theories has advanced our understanding of the complexities of suicidal behavior (Díaz-Oliván et al., 2021; O'Connor & Nock, 2014). These theories examine different aspects of suicide's etiopathogenesis. They are grounded in extensive research that suggests that suicide risk arises from the dynamic interplay of biological, psychological, environmental, social, and cultural factors over time (Knipe et al., 2022; Turecki & Brent, 2016).

Despite progress in identifying risk factors and developing theoretical models of suicidal behavior, significant challenges persist in integrating these factors into comprehensive frameworks. Many theoretical models have yet to provide specific markers of suicide risk (Li et al., 2022) and often fail to offer clinically helpful tools for managing suicidal behavior (Carter & Spittal, 2018; Hawton et al., 2022). A meta-analysis spanning five decades of research revealed that our ability to predict suicidal behavior is only slightly better than chance (Franklin et al., 2017). Current suicide risk assessment tools lack sufficient accuracy to be clinically valuable due to

Á. Jiménez-Molina (✉)
Faculty of Psychology and Humanities, Universidad San Sebastián,
Santiago, RM - Santiago, Chile

Millennium Institute for Research in Depression and Personality (MIDAP), Santiago, Chile

Nucleus to Improve the Mental Health of Adolescents and Youths (Imhay), Santiago, Chile
e-mail: alvaro.jimenez@uss.cl

Á. Jiménez-Molina, V. Martínez (eds.), *New Perspectives on Suicidal Behavior*, Depression and Personality, https://doi.org/10.1007/978-3-031-96037-6_2

their low predictive validity, sensitivity, and specificity (Runeson et al., 2017). For example, over 90% of individuals classified as high-risk do not subsequently exhibit suicidal behavior (Carter et al., 2017). As a result, our ability to prevent suicide remains as limited today as it was 50 years ago (Fox et al., 2020).

A decade ago, the DSM-5 introduced suicidal behavior disorder (SBD) as a condition for further study, which considers previous suicide attempts and represents a lifetime risk (American Psychiatric Association, 2013). However, this category has sparked controversy (Schuck et al., 2019). While a previous suicide attempt is a well-known risk factor, most individuals who attempt suicide do not die by suicide. Similarly, although mental illness significantly raises suicide risk, most individuals with mental illness do not die by suicide or attempt it.

Understanding suicidal behavior remains challenging due to several key factors. First, individuals who die by suicide cannot be evaluated psychologically, and they may differ significantly from those who attempt suicide or experience suicidal thoughts. Additionally, because only a tiny fraction of those who think about suicide attempt it—and even fewer die by suicide—large sample sizes are needed to study suicide risk (O'Connor & Portzky, 2018). The field also lacks common terminology (Goodfellow et al., 2019), and many risk factors, such as early adversity, are too usual to distinguish between individuals effectively. Suicidal crises are typically temporary, and fluctuating (Rudd, 2006), yet risk factors are often assessed statically rather than dynamically, leading to an incomplete understanding of the complex interactions that lead to suicide (Franklin et al., 2017; O'Connor & Portzky, 2018).

Undoubtedly, these challenges contribute to the slow progress in understanding suicidal behavior. However, a significant part of the problem likely arises from the limitations of existing theoretical models and the traditional methods used in psychology to develop and evaluate these theories. As a result of these theoretical issues, suicidality research often repeats similar studies, focusing on the same factors associated with suicidal behavior and testing the same hypotheses using similar approaches (Hjelmeland, 2016). In this context, this chapter offers an overview of key findings in the psychology of suicidal behavior, presents major integrative theoretical models and their associated challenges, and provides a critical perspective on developing theoretical frameworks in suicidology.

2.2 Theoretical Models of Suicidal Behavior

Several psychological models have been developed to explain how various factors combine to increase suicide risk, with a distinction between first- and second-generation theories of suicidal behavior. Among the first-generation theories are the psychodynamic theory, Shneidman's theory of "psychache," and Baumeister's escape from self-theory.

The psychodynamic theory posits that the suicidal process begins with the unconscious loss of a love object. When unable to fulfill their need for love and attachment, the individual redirects their anger inward, potentially leading to self-destructive behaviors (Goldblatt, 2014). Shneidman's theory (1993, 1998) conceptualizes suicide as an attempt to escape overwhelming psychological pain caused by unmet needs. This pain, called "psychache," arises from intense emotions such as shame, guilt, humiliation, loneliness, or anguish and is seen as the primary driver of suicidal behavior. According to Shneidman, individuals who die by suicide are in profound emotional distress, though they may not necessarily have a clinical mental illness.

Likewise, Baumeister's escape from self theory (1990) views suicide as the culmination of a process in which the individual seeks to escape from themselves and reality. This process begins with the perception of failing to meet expectations, leading to self-criticism and negative self-awareness, accompanied by feelings of incompetence, lack of affection, anxiety, and depression. As this state intensifies, the individual becomes narrowly focused on the present, feels powerless, and adopts irrational attitudes that decide to take their own life more likely.

First-generation theories, grounded mainly in the clinical judgment of professionals, often focus on specific risk factors for suicidal behavior. However, they failed to differentiate the conditions that lead to suicidal ideation from those that result in suicide attempts or death by suicide. Additionally, they did not account for why most individuals who experience suicidal thoughts never proceed to attempt suicide.

Second-generation theories, emerging since the 2000s within the "ideation-to-action" model, focus on the factors that mediate the transition from suicidal thoughts to suicidal behavior. These theories propose that while the processes underlying suicidal ideation and suicidal attempt may overlap, they are distinct and thus require separate explanations (Klonsky et al., 2017; O'Connor & Nock, 2014). By offering this new perspective, second-generation theories have significantly advanced the study of suicide, paving the way for more targeted therapeutic and preventive interventions.

Three models stand out within this framework: the interpersonal-psychological theory, the integrated motivational-volitional model, and the three-step theory (Joiner, 2007; Klonsky & May, 2015; O'Connor, 2011; Van Orden et al., 2010). While each of these theories emphasizes different factors contributing to suicidal ideation and behavior, they all share a common perspective that has profoundly shaped the current understanding of the suicidal process: (1) suicidal thoughts and behaviors arise from the convergence of aversive emotional and cognitive states; (2) they surface when other coping mechanisms fail to relieve unbearable psychological distress; and (3) suicide is seen as a means of escaping this overwhelming suffering.

2.2.1 The Interpersonal Psychological Theory of Suicide

The interpersonal psychological theory (IPT) of suicide posits that people die by suicide because they have both the desire and the capability to do so. The coexistence of high levels of perceived burdensomeness (i.e., feeling like a burden to others) and low levels of belongingness (i.e., feeling alienated or not belonging), along with hopelessness that these states will not change, leads to the development of suicidal desire (Joiner, 2007). Suicidal desire is a necessary but not sufficient cause for a suicide attempt. The "acquired capability" for suicide relates to the ability to carry out the act, which includes a reduced fear of death and an increased tolerance for physical pain (Van Orden et al., 2010).

The IPT suggests that thwarted belongingness is a multidimensional and dynamic cognitive-affective state composed of two main factors: loneliness and the absence of reciprocally caring relationships. Loneliness is the perception of having few meaningful social connections or lacking satisfactory interactions. The absence of reciprocally caring relationships refers to the lack of relationships characterized by mutual care and support, manifesting in feelings of not being a support to others or not having someone to turn to in times of need. This theory distinguishes itself from previous theories by proposing that an unmet "need to belong" is the specific interpersonal need involved in the emergence of the desire to die. Thwarted belongingness does not imply the lack of human connections; perceived burdensomeness can exist even without significant relationships. Satisfying the need to belong is not simply achieved through the presence of human connections.

According to the IPT, perceived burdensomeness comprises two dimensions of interpersonal functioning: on the one hand, the beliefs that one is so defective that one becomes a burden to others ("My family would be better off without me"); on the other hand, self-hostile cognitions that result in low self-esteem or self-blame ("I am useless"). This aspect is evident in risk factors such as severe physical illnesses, the stress caused by unemployment, or family conflicts that can increase the perception of being a burden to others. This dimension can be observed in statements in suicide notes or in the case of adolescent suicidal behavior, where perceptions of being expendable within the family are particularly crucial (Van Orden et al., 2010).

Traditional models assumed that the risk of suicide increases with the intensity of suicidal desire. However, the IPT argues that the desire to die is not sufficient to carry out a suicide attempt. Many people do not attempt suicide because they fear it and the associated physical pain. According to IPT, the acquired capability for suicide is linked to a reduced fear of death and a greater tolerance for physical pain. This capability can be developed through habituation and repeated exposure to painful and/or distressing experiences, such as childhood adversity, trauma, and violence. Continuous exposure to these experiences increases pain tolerance, enabling a person to engage in increasingly lethal forms of self-harm. In this context, pain tolerance is viewed as a dimensional phenomenon related to suicide methods. The common factor in all methods of suicide is the cognitive assessment that the pain involved is tolerable, which can explain why suicide methods are generally not substituted.

In summary, the IPT suggests that thwarted belongingness, perceived burdensomeness, and acquired capability are distinct yet interrelated constructs. The same etiological processes or mechanisms underlie all forms of suicidal behavior, although they are not necessarily the only pathways. The confluence of these conditions is rare, explaining why most individuals with a risk factor do not attempt suicide (Van Orden et al., 2010).

2.2.2 *Integrated Motivational-Volitional Model of Suicidal Behavior*

The integrated motivational-volitional (IMV) model conceptualizes suicidal behavior as a phenomenon that develops through premotivational, motivational, and volitional phases rather than merely being a consequence of mental disorders (O'Connor, 2011; O'Connor & Kirtley, 2018). This model comprises three distinct phases.

First, the premotivational phase outlines the biopsychosocial context in which vulnerability factors and triggering events influence suicidal ideation and behavior. Biological and genetic vulnerabilities, combined with life stressors like childhood adversities, set the stage for developing suicidal ideation. In this phase, the model integrates the diathesis-stress perspective, suggesting that combining individual vulnerabilities—such as personality traits or socio-environmental factors—and stressors increases the likelihood of an adverse psychological reaction.

Second, the motivational phase focuses on psychological processes leading to suicidal ideation and intent. The model posits that the strongest predictor of suicidal behavior is the individual's intention or motivation. While a sense of belonging and perceived burdensomeness is central to the IPT, the IMV model highlights feelings of defeat, humiliation, and entrapment by life circumstances as key predictors. Premotivational vulnerabilities, such as socially prescribed perfectionism, increase sensitivity to defeat, with entrapment bridging defeat and suicidal ideation.

Finally, the volitional phase identifies "volitional moderators" that increase the likelihood of transitioning from suicidal ideation to action. These moderators include access to lethal means, exposure to others' suicidal behavior, planning, impulsivity, and past suicidal behavior. While the ITS emphasizes acquired capability, the IMV model views it as one of several factors that increase the likelihood of a suicide attempt. The model suggests that repeated distress strengthens the association between distress and suicidal ideation, making suicidal thoughts more readily activated and translating intention into action more rapidly.

2.2.3 *The Three-Step Theory*

The three-step theory (3ST) aims to explain suicidal behavior through the interaction of four key factors: pain, hopelessness, connection, and the capability for suicide, within a three-phase process (Klonsky & May, 2015).

According to this theory, the first step toward suicidal ideation begins with pain, generally referring to psychological or emotional pain. Although this pain can diminish the desire to live, it is not enough to trigger suicidal behavior. A person experiencing pain but holding onto hope that the situation will improve is likely to focus on the future rather than consider suicide. However, when pain is combined with hopelessness, the individual is more likely to contemplate suicide as an option. Unlike theories that focus solely on pain or hopelessness, such as Shneidman's (1993), the 3ST holds that it is the combination of both factors that leads to suicidal ideation.

The second step emphasizes the role of connection, which can be with other people, a job, a project, or any sense of purpose that keeps a person engaged in life. Unlike the IPT, which conceptualizes thwarted belongingness as a critical risk component, 3ST argues that suicidal ideation can develop without disrupted connections. Thus, connections should be seen as a protective rather than a risk factor. If the connection to life outweighs the experience of pain or hopelessness, the individual will not experience an escalation of suicidal ideation. However, if this connection is absent or weaker than the pain and hopelessness, the person will develop an active desire to end their life (Klonsky & May, 2015). From this perspective, some traditional risk factors, such as depression, self-criticism, or interpersonal losses, are relevant to suicidal ideation insofar as they are associated with pain, hopelessness, or connection.

The third step considers that the progression from ideation to suicide attempts is facilitated by dispositional, acquired, and practical factors. While 3ST agrees with the IPT that the key determinant for a suicide attempt is the individual's capability to carry it out, it expands the notion of capability into three categories: dispositional capability refers to genetically driven variables, such as pain sensitivity; acquired capability refers to habituation to pain and fear of death related to experiences like abuse or self-injury; while practical capability involves concrete factors that facilitate a suicide attempt, such as access to lethal means.

Table 2.1 summarizes some of the main theories of suicidal behavior, and the intervention focuses derived from them.

Table 2.1 Main theoretical models of suicidal behavior

Theoretical model	Description	Intervention focus
Psychological pain/"psychache" (Shneidman, 1993)	Suicide is a result of psychological pain (psychache) perceived as intolerable, unmanageable, or unending. This pain stems from the frustration of basic psychological needs such as love, acceptance, belonging, control, and achievement.	The therapeutic focus is aimed at alleviating the pain caused by unmet psychological needs (hopelessness, frustration, deteriorated self-esteem, and the rupture of significant relationships) and at reducing the tendency to act impulsively.
Escape from self (Baumeister, 1990)	Suicide is understood as an attempt to escape aversive self-awareness, which arises when a person realizes that their life does not meet their expectations, leading to negative self-evaluation. To cope with this pain, individuals turn to cognitive deconstruction, a mental process aimed at avoiding this painful self-awareness. This can lead to emotional emptiness, an increase in negative emotions, and a mental state of lowered inhibition, ultimately increasing the risk of suicide.	The therapeutic approach focuses on the psychological pain stemming from negative self-awareness and the development of alternative coping strategies for the medium to long term. It aims to foster greater tolerance and regulation of aversive internal states while addressing the underlying causes by confronting them rather than attempting to escape from them.

(continued)

Table 2.1 (continued)

Theoretical model	Description	Intervention focus
Cognitive model (Wenzel et al., 2009)	Suicide is associated with a cognitive functioning style characterized by rigidity (schemas), dichotomous thinking, confirmation bias (distortions), and hopelessness (negative future expectations).	The therapeutic approach focuses on changing cognitive functioning and processes, particularly harmful belief systems about oneself and others (e.g., seeing oneself as unlovable or perceiving others as abandoning).
Fluid vulnerability (Rudd, 2006)	The "suicidal mode" manifests across cognitive, emotional, physiological, and behavioral domains and is driven by four core beliefs: feeling unloved, helplessness, low distress tolerance, and the perception of being a burden. Cognitive rigidity, or the inability to adapt to new situations, is a key feature in the cognitive domain. Emotional dysregulation further impairs the ability to sustain goal-directed behaviors during periods of distress. As the body cannot maintain a heightened state of arousal indefinitely, this suicidal mode is temporary, and the risk of suicide fluctuates over time.	The therapeutic approach focuses on core beliefs that increase suicide risk, along with emotion regulation and reducing vulnerability during crises.
Stress-diathesis model (Mann & Rizk, 2020)	Suicide is linked to epigenetic factors, such as traumatic experiences in childhood or adulthood, combined with genetic vulnerability. When factors like stress and triggering events are added, a synergistic effect is generated, increasing the risk of suicidal behavior.	The therapeutic approach aims to reduce vulnerability by addressing risk factors such as impulsivity, emotional dysregulation, and rigid or hopeless thinking. It focuses on strengthening coping skills, improving problem-solving, and increasing tolerance for emotional distress, reducing susceptibility through cognitive and emotional changes, while managing external stressors.
Interpersonal psychological theory (Joiner, 2007)	The risk of suicide arises from the interaction of three key factors: the perception of being a burden, the feeling of isolation or lack of belonging, and the acquired capability to carry out the suicidal act.	The therapeutic approach aims to help the individual reassess their self-esteem and relationships more realistically and positively, fostering a sense of belonging and reducing emotional isolation. It also focuses on addressing desensitization to pain while promoting strategies to manage impulses and limit access to lethal means.

(continued)

Table 2.1 (continued)

Theoretical model	Description	Intervention focus
Integrated motivational-volitional model (O'Connor, 2011)	The suicidal process is divided into three phases: premotivational, motivational (where suicidal ideation and intent develop), and volitional (where the behavior is carried out). Feelings of defeat and entrapment act as key moderating factors, influencing the transition from ideation to action and increasing the risk of suicide.	The therapeutic approach focuses on addressing feelings of defeat, hopelessness, and entrapment while simultaneously working to reduce impulsivity.
Three-step theory (3ST) (Klonsky & May, 2015)	Suicidal thoughts arise from the combination of psychological pain and hopelessness, while a sense of connection serves as a protective factor against the intensification of suicidal ideation. The transition from ideation to suicide attempts is facilitated by dispositional, acquired, and practical factors that increase the capacity to confront pain and fear with the intent of ending one's life.	The therapeutic approach is focused on psychological pain, hopelessness, and the sense of connection.
Control without awareness (Macintyre et al., 2021)	Suicidal behavior is understood as a strategy to regain a sense of control in response to feelings of entrapment and defeat and to avoid painful memories and conflict between significant life goals.	The therapeutic approach focuses on restoring control by increasing awareness of the conflicts between life goals.
Suicide crisis syndrome (SCS) (Schuck et al., 2019)	Suicide crisis is characterized by intense emotions and cognitive disturbances, particularly a sense of entrapment, often accompanied by dissociative experiences. These states, characterized by uncontrollable fear and repetitive ruminative thoughts, intensify feelings of despair and hopelessness, making suicide seem like an escape from unbearable emotional pain.	The therapeutic approach focuses on the emotional and cognitive states that accompany a suicidal crisis, aiming to relieve the feeling of entrapment and loss of cognitive control. Emotional regulation techniques are used to manage panic and dissociation while working to address social withdrawal and repetitive thoughts related to hopelessness.

2.3 Implications for Clinical Practice and Prevention

Theoretical models should not only aid in understanding the complex interplay of factors that elevate suicide risk but also offer a practical framework for evaluating, identifying etiological connections, setting intervention targets, and preventing suicidal behavior. The psychological domains identified as significant in various theories of suicide include psychological pain and the skills to regulate it (Klonsky &

May, 2015; Shneidman, 1993), self-perceptions and feelings toward oneself (Baumeister, 1990; Joiner, 2007; Rudd, 2006), interpersonal connections and sense of belonging (Joiner, 2007; Klonsky & May, 2015; Rudd, 2006; Van Orden et al., 2010), hopelessness (Joiner, 2007; Klonsky & May, 2015; O'Connor, 2011), and feelings of defeat and entrapment (O'Connor, 2011).

From the perspective of the IPT, clinical intervention should focus on reducing thwarted belongingness and perceived burdensomeness, as these are dynamic and amenable to change. In contrast, acquired capability is more stable (Van Orden et al., 2010). Similarly, the IMV model suggests that interventions and routine clinical care should be tailored to the model phase in which the person is situated, focusing on modifiable factors such as perceptions of defeat and entrapment (O'Connor, 2011).

The previously presented theoretical models have received varying empirical support (Díaz-Oliván et al., 2021; O'Connor & Kirtley, 2018; O'Connor & Nock, 2014). For instance, a network analysis of cross-sectional data from a sample of Scottish adults indicated that a central component of each theory (IPT: perceived burdensomeness; IMV: internal entrapment) was strongly related to suicidal ideation, while other central components (IPT: thwarted belongingness; IMV: defeat, external entrapment) did not show strong direct relationships with suicidal ideation, suggesting they might function as moderators or mediators (De Beurs et al., 2019).

"Ideation-to-action" models (IPT, IMV, 3ST) represent a significant advance in the conceptualization and research of suicidal behavior. However, several limitations in clinical and preventive contexts warrant attention. For instance, these models often present a linear structure of the suicidal process, beginning with the desire to die and culminating in suicide. Typically organized around groups of factors (predisposing and precipitating), this structure does not always capture the phenomenon's complexity or its recurrence over time. Additionally, these models have been criticized for relying on a risk assessment framework centered on self-reported suicidal ideation, which has proven to be limited in effectively identifying risk in clinical settings. Explicit suicidal ideation can last less than 10 min before an attempt, and only a minority of those who die by suicide exhibit such ideation beforehand (Schuck et al., 2019).

Moreover, a significant challenge for practitioners applying these models in treatment is their limited clinical relevance. It has been suggested that current theoretical models fail to adequately account for the dynamic nature of suicide risk, with an overemphasis on prediction at the expense of prevention and clinical management (Hawton et al., 2022). In contrast, given that psychological states are highly variable and create uncertainty about their progression, clinical approaches should prioritize building a strong therapeutic alliance (Hawton et al., 2022).

In prevention, it is essential to deepen the understanding of protective factors and barriers to help-seeking. However, protective factors have received insufficient theoretical attention. Although elements such as optimism, resilience, and social connection have been identified (Zortea et al., 2020), the mechanisms underlying recovery from suicidal thoughts and behaviors remain poorly understood.

A comprehensive theory of suicide must also address demographic differences in suicide rates, which vary by gender, age, and culture. For instance, theoretical models should help explain the "gender paradox" (where men die by suicide more often, yet women make more attempts). However, current models suggest that the underlying psychology of suicidal behavior is similar in men and women (Bennett et al., 2023) without accounting for how gender-specific factors—such as the influence of cultural norms on emotional experience and regulation—affect suicidal behavior.

2.4 Methodological Challenges in Suicide Research

The theoretical models of suicide result from a synthesis of various methodological approaches. Epidemiological studies examine the associations between suicide rates and various social factors, such as economic circumstances and social cohesion, by comparing different populations (Chandler, 2020; Stuckler & Basu, 2013; Wray et al., 2011). Biological studies suggest that suicidal behavior results from a combination of biological predispositions and psychosocial stressors, investigating genetic and neurobiological factors in specific populations, such as serotonin dysregulation and reduced activity in the prefrontal cortex (Mann, 2003; Mann & Rizk, 2020) or transdiagnostic dimensions according to RDoC domains, such as deficiencies in stress response systems (Glenn et al., 2018). Psychological autopsy studies retrospectively determine the antecedents of suicides through interviews with close informants and the examination of medical records (Cavanagh et al., 2003), dividing the causes of suicide between individual psychology and the interpersonal environment, often emphasizing the assumed causal role of mental disorders (Hjelmeland et al., 2012). Qualitative studies aim to understand the meaning of suicidal acts, suggesting that structural and psychological influences should be interpreted in the sociocultural context (Cover, 2016; Hjelmeland & Knizek, 2010).

To enhance the understanding of suicidal behavior, as well as clinical practices and prevention strategies, suicide research must embrace multimethod approaches and explanatory pluralism, integrating factors and mechanisms across multiple levels. In this regard, there is a need for longitudinal designs, as most studies are cross-sectional (O'Connor & Portzky, 2018). Longitudinal research is crucial for establishing causality over time and determining whether identified variables contribute to suicidal ideation and attempts rather than being a consequence of these behaviors. Additionally, it is essential to clarify the time frames in which risk factors lead to suicidal ideation and attempts.

Traditional statistical techniques in psychology, such as analysis of variance or regression analysis, often focus on identifying risk factors but offer a limited view of the relationships between these factors. Network analysis and other emerging techniques provide new opportunities better to understand the complex interplay between multiple interrelated variables. These tools enable the comparison of the relative importance of key factors linked to suicidal ideation and behavior, combining predictive approaches with a deeper exploration of the relationships between various risk factors, which can help identify more effective treatment targets (De Beurs et al., 2019). However, despite their potential, research in this field remains limited.

Since suicide is an intentional and deliberate act, it carries a meaning that is rooted in a cultural context. Additionally, many people live with various risk factors for years before deciding to take their own lives. To understand the significance these factors, hold for each individual, it is essential to analyze them concerning their lived experience. Therefore, to not only *explain* but, more importantly, to *understand* suicidal behavior, we need more and better qualitative research (Hjelmeland & Knizek, 2010).

In recent years, the use of digital technologies and smartphones has allowed for real-time tracking of participants' thoughts, feelings, and behaviors, demonstrating significant variability in suicidal ideation among individuals (O'Connor & Portzky, 2018). Additionally, recent studies have explored the potential of machine learning (ML) in detecting, monitoring, and supporting individuals at risk of suicide, showing high predictive value and sensitivity for suicide risk cases (Grimland et al., 2024). A meta-analysis found that ML models perform satisfactorily in predicting suicidal ideation and attempts, with reasonable specificity and moderate sensitivity (Kusuma et al., 2022). A literature review reported that natural language processing (NLP) methods are generally accurate and robust in detecting suicidal thoughts or behaviors, outperforming human interpretations and symptom-based identification methods (Young et al., 2023). These findings suggest that NLP could enhance suicide risk detection. However, further research is needed to integrate these artificial intelligence (AI) models with psychological theories and explore their utility in developing and testing various theoretical models.

2.5 Theoretical Challenges in Suicide Research

In psychology, research often emphasizes a methodological approach focused on testing (accepting or rejecting) empirical hypotheses, dedicating less time to the conceptual work necessary for constructing theories about processes and mechanisms (Borsboom et al., 2021). However, theories are intended to provide understanding through creative explanations and are epistemologically prior to any empirical testing (Borsboom et al., 2021; van Rooij & Baggio, 2020). While it would be naive to expect a single theory to explain all cases of suicide, theories are valuable if they guide us in identifying what is worth investigating.

It can be argued that the relative stagnation in contemporary suicide research is not solely an empirical issue that can be resolved by generating more data but may also be linked to a more profound theoretical crisis. On the one hand, the diversity of approaches in suicidology leads to "incommensurability" (Maung, 2020), which complicates empirical comparisons between theoretical models and limits their conceptual integration. This is an epistemological issue that requires theoretical reflection on the conceptual foundations underlying these different approaches.

On the other hand, many studies embark on a disorganized search for potential risk factors, lacking a solid theoretical foundation or a coherent conceptual framework (Hjelmeland, 2016). Although research continues to identify more variables involved in suicidal behavior, knowledge about the synergistic effects between different theoretical constructs and the mechanisms underlying suicidal behavior remains very limited. While there is no shortage of theoretical models proposing principles based on the interaction of multiple risk factors (Díaz-Oliván et al., 2021), there is a risk that clinical practice and research become driven by disconnected empirical findings organized around fragmented risk factors. Although there has been significant progress in the technical refinement (e.g., statistical) of studies, this is insufficient to transform a set of variables into a theoretical model (of processes and mechanisms) that explains psychological phenomena rather than merely capturing patterns in the data (van Rooij & Baggio, 2020).

This situation leads to at least two undesirable consequences: first, we lack a solid understanding of how different phenomena relate to one another; second, we continue replicating the same studies and testing the same hypotheses. Indeed, it has been criticized that suicidality research no longer formulates new theories but has become fixated on replicating results from studies examining the same psychological, epidemiological, and neurobiological factors associated with suicide (Hjelmeland, 2016; Lester, 2000). This is partly because the factors studied are often selected based on their availability in commonly used assessment scales or predefined diagnostic criteria. However, repetitive studies on already known risk factors do not provide helpful knowledge.

Another theoretical challenge in suicide research relates to the nature of theoretical models. Both explicitly and implicitly, these models in psychology present different approaches to the levels of explanation and the key mechanisms involved in understanding the causes of suicidal behavior. To improve the understanding of suicidal behavior, a theory needs to be comprehensive (able to explain both suicidal ideation and suicide attempts) and precise (allowing for scientific falsifiability and clinical utility). This demand for intelligibility aims to make suicidal behavior rationally comprehensible. The problem with this approach is that in psychology, we often encounter "causation" that does not appear rational, and the notion of a mechanism is notably obscure (Campbell, 2015). Does this mean we should abandon the idea of a mechanism as a set of levers underlying suicidal behavior? One way to address this problem is to acknowledge that a "mechanism" cannot be explained without referring to the idea of a counterfactual under an intervention (Campbell, 2015). From this viewpoint, the theoretical question involves identifying variables whose interventions result in changes to the outcome variable, in this case, suicidal behavior. While this approach could open new pathways for suicide research, it also introduces significant ethical and methodological challenges.

2.6 A Critical Theory of Suicide

Some of the most compelling theoretical and methodological debates in contemporary suicide research are emerging within the field of critical suicidology. This perspective challenges a fundamental premise of modern suicidology: that suicidal behavior is inherently individual and pathological and, therefore, primarily a medical issue (White et al., 2016). Critical suicidology questions the prevailing assumption that most people who die by suicide—up to 90% (Cavanagh et al., 2003)—suffer from a diagnosable mental disorder, which has led traditional suicidology to focus disproportionately on pathology and deficit. Instead, it argues that suicide should be understood as a phenomenon deeply rooted in socio-cultural and political contexts, as no suicidal act occurs in isolation from the prevailing norms and values of a cultural community (Cover, 2016; White et al., 2016). In doing so, critical suicidology challenges key assumptions underpinning dominant theoretical models of suicidal behavior.

While not denying the role mental disorders can play in suicidal behavior, critical suicidology suggests that they should be understood contextually, arguing that framing certain types of distress in terms of psychiatric illness diverts attention from the social circumstances enabling these types of distress (Hjelmeland & Knizek, 2017). This is not merely an empirical disagreement about the exaggerated proportion of suicides associated with mental disorders (Hjelmeland et al., 2012) but also a fundamental disagreement about different ways of understanding mental disorders and suicide (Hjelmeland & Knizek, 2017; Maung, 2020). Additionally, critical suicidology is concerned that conventional suicidology's tendency to attribute suicide to mental disorders reflects and reinforces a hegemony that privileges a Western biomedical approach to suffering, mainly when Western psychiatric concepts are applied to people from non-Western communities or those experiencing various forms of social suffering or structural violence (Cover, 2016; White et al., 2016).

Émile Durkheim's pioneering research was crucial in emphasizing the social dimensions of suicide. Rather than focusing on individual psychology, Durkheim explained suicide as a broader social phenomenon, highlighting how variations in suicide rates are linked to the structure of social relationships (Durkheim, 2015). Since Durkheim's foundational work, numerous studies have shown that suicide rates are dynamic and highly responsive to social, political, and economic conditions (Duarte & Jiménez-Molina, 2023; Stuckler & Basu, 2013; Wray et al., 2011).

In recent decades, various approaches have highlighted the importance of social factors in suicidal behaviors, incorporating concepts such as social determinants of health, social suffering, and structural violence (Chandler, 2020). However, major theoretical models have struggled to conceptualize and integrate the sociocultural dimensions of suicidal behavior. It can be argued that these models view "the social" as merely an environment surrounding individuals, a collection of individual risk factors (socioeconomic status, childhood adversity, education, discrimination, unemployment, among others), and a predetermined set of attributes to be measured or modified. In doing so, the social is understood apart from the daily practices and historical-cultural conditions that shape individual and collective life, overlooking the inherent *sociability* of the social (Jiménez-Molina, 2018). In public mental health, this approach generates a perspective that promotes policies focused on "social deficits" and targets specific groups rather than addressing broader social structures (Bemme & Béhague, 2024). Critical suicidology, however, asserts that social factors do not just influence suicidal behaviors, but rather that such behaviors are inherently social phenomena. This perspective undoubtedly presents challenges for the development of new theoretical models of suicidal behavior.

Acknowledgments This manuscript was supported by ANID—Millennium Science Initiative Program—AIM23_0002 and NCS2021_081 and by ANID—FONIS SA23I0181.

References

American Psychiatric Association. (2013). *Diagnostic and statistical manual of mental disorders* (5th ed.). American Psychiatric Publishing.

Baumeister, R. F. (1990). Suicide as escape from self. *Psychological Review, 97*(1), 90–113. https://doi.org/10.1037/0033-295X.97.1.90

Bemme, D., & Béhague, D. (2024). Theorising the social in mental health research and action: A call for more inclusivity and accountability. *Social Psychiatry and Psychiatric Epidemiology, 59*(3), 403–408. https://doi.org/10.1007/s00127-024-02632-2

Bennett, S., Robb, K. A., Zortea, T. C., Dickson, A., Richardson, C., & O'Connor, R. C. (2023). Male suicide risk and recovery factors: A systematic review and qualitative metasynthesis of two decades of research. *Psychological Bulletin, 149*(7–8), 371–417. https://doi.org/10.1037/bul0000397

Borsboom, D., van der Maas, H. L. J., Dalege, J., Kievit, R. A., & Haig, B. D. (2021). Theory construction methodology: A practical framework for building theories in psychology. *Perspectives on Psychological Science: A Journal of the Association for Psychological Science, 16*(4), 756–766. https://doi.org/10.1177/1745691620969647

Campbell, J. (2015). Causation and mechanism in psychiatry. In K. Fulford, M. Davies, et al. (Eds.), *The Oxford handbook of philosophy and psychiatry* (pp. 935–949). Oxford University Press.

Carter, G., Milner, A., McGill, K., Pirkis, J., Kapur, N., & Spittal, M. J. (2017). Predicting suicidal behaviours using clinical instruments: Systematic review and meta-analysis of positive predictive values for risk scales. *The British Journal of Psychiatry: the Journal of Mental Science, 210*(6), 387–395. https://doi.org/10.1192/bjp.bp.116.182717

Carter, G., & Spittal, M. J. (2018). Suicide risk assessment: Risk stratification is not accurate enough to be clinically useful and alternative approaches are needed. *Crisis: The Journal of Crisis Intervention and Suicide Prevention, 39*(4), 229–234. https://doi.org/10.1027/0227-5910/a000558

Cavanagh, J. T., Carson, A. J., Sharpe, M., & Lawrie, S. M. (2003). Psychological autopsy studies of suicide: A systematic review. *Psychological Medicine, 33*(3), 395–405. https://doi.org/10.1017/s0033291702006943

Chandler, A. (2020). Socioeconomic inequalities of suicide: Sociological and psychological intersections. *European Journal of Social Theory, 23*(1), 33–51. https://doi.org/10.1177/1368431018804154

Cover, R. (2016). Suicides of the marginalised: Cultural approaches to suicide, minorities and relationality. *Cultural Studies Review, 22*(2), 90–113. https://doi.org/10.5130/csr.v22i2.4708

De Beurs, D., Fried, E. I., Wetherall, K., Cleare, S., O' Connor, D. B., Ferguson, E., O'Carroll, R. E., & O'Connor, R. C. (2019). Exploring the psychology of suicidal ideation: A theory driven

network analysis. *Behaviour Research and Therapy, 120*, 103419. https://doi.org/10.1016/j.brat.2019.103419
Díaz-Oliván, I., Porras-Segovia, A., Barrigón, M., Jiménez-Muñoz, L., & Baca-García, E. (2021). Theoretical models of suicidal behaviour: A systematic review and narrative synthesis. *European Journal of Psychiatry, 35*(3), 181–192. https://doi.org/10.1016/j.ejpsy.2021.02.002
Duarte, F., & Jiménez-Molina, Á. (2023). Suicide and quarantine during the COVID-19 pandemic: Do we know everything? *Social Science & Medicine, 309*, 115253. https://doi.org/10.1016/j.socscimed.2022.115253
Durkheim, É. (1897/2015). *El suicidio*. Akal.
Fox, K. R., Huang, X., Guzmán, E. M., Funsch, K. M., Cha, C. B., Ribeiro, J. D., & Franklin, J. C. (2020). Interventions for suicide and self-injury: A meta-analysis of randomized controlled trials across nearly 50 years of research. *Psychological Bulletin, 146*(12), 1117–1145. https://doi.org/10.1037/bul0000305
Franklin, J. C., Ribeiro, J. D., Fox, K. R., Bentley, K. H., Kleiman, E. M., Huang, X., Musacchio, K. M., Jaroszewski, A. C., Chang, B. P., & Nock, M. K. (2017). Risk factors for suicidal thoughts and behaviors: A meta-analysis of 50 years of research. *Psychological Bulletin, 143*(2), 187–232. https://doi.org/10.1037/bul0000084
Glenn, C. R., Kleiman, E. M., Cha, C. B., Deming, C. A., Franklin, J. C., & Nock, M. K. (2018). Understanding suicide risk within the Research Domain Criteria (RDoC) framework: A meta-analytic review. *Depression and Anxiety, 35*(1), 65–88. https://doi.org/10.1002/da.22686
Goldblatt, M. (2014). Psychodynamics of suicide. In M. Nock (Ed.), *The Oxford handbook of suicide and self-injury* (pp. 255–264). Oxford University Press.
Goodfellow, B., Kõlves, K., & de Leo, D. (2019). Contemporary definitions of suicidal behavior: A systematic literature review. *Suicide & Life-Threatening Behavior, 49*(2), 488–504. https://doi.org/10.1111/sltb.12457
Grimland, M., Benatov, J., Yeshayahu, H., Izmaylov, D., Segal, A., Gal, K., & Levi-Belz, Y. (2024). Predicting suicide risk in real-time crisis hotline chats integrating machine learning with psychological factors: Exploring the black box. *Suicide & Life-Threatening Behavior, 54*(3), 416–424. https://doi.org/10.1111/sltb.13056
Hawton, K., Lascelles, K., Pitman, A., Gilbert, S., & Silverman, M. (2022). Assessment of suicide risk in mental health practice: Shifting from prediction to therapeutic assessment, formulation, and risk management. *The Lancet. Psychiatry, 9*(11), 922–928. https://doi.org/10.1016/S2215-0366(22)00232-2
Hjelmeland, H. (2016). A critical look at current suicide research. In J. White, I. Marsh, M. Kral, & J. Morris (Eds.), *Critical suicidology: Transforming suicide research and prevention for the 21st century* (pp. 135–154). UBC Press.
Hjelmeland, H., Dieserud, G., Dyregrov, K., Knizek, B. L., & Leenaars, A. A. (2012). Psychological autopsy studies as diagnostic tools: Are they methodologically flawed? *Death Studies, 36*(7), 605–626. https://doi.org/10.1080/07481187.2011.584015
Hjelmeland, H., & Knizek, B. L. (2010). Why we need qualitative research in suicidology. *Suicide & Life-Threatening Behavior, 40*(1), 74–80. https://doi.org/10.1521/suli.2010.40.1.74
Hjelmeland, H., & Knizek, B. L. (2017). Suicide and mental disorders: A discourse of politics, power, and vested interests. *Death Studies, 41*(8), 481–492. https://doi.org/10.1080/07481187.2017.1332905
Jiménez-Molina, A. (2018). *L'adolescence mutilée: Grammaires de la souffrance au Chili et en France*. Doctoral thesis, Université Paris Cité.
Joiner, T. E. (2007). *Why people die by suicide*. Harvard University Press.
Klonsky, E. D., & May, A. M. (2015). The Three-Step Theory (3ST): A new theory of suicide rooted in the "ideation-to-action" framework. *International Journal of Cognitive Therapy, 8*(2), 114–129. https://doi.org/10.1521/ijct.2015.8.2.114
Klonsky, E. D., Qiu, T., & Saffer, B. Y. (2017). Recent advances in differentiating suicide attempters from suicide ideators. *Current Opinion in Psychiatry, 30*(1), 15–20. https://doi.org/10.1097/YCO.0000000000000294

Knipe, D., Padmanathan, P., Newton-Howes, G., Chan, L. F., & Kapur, N. (2022). Suicide and self-harm. *Lancet (London, England), 399*(10338), 1903–1916. https://doi.org/10.1016/S0140-6736(22)00173-8

Kusuma, K., Larsen, M., Quiroz, J. C., Gillies, M., Burnett, A., Qian, J., & Torok, M. (2022). The performance of machine learning models in predicting suicidal ideation, attempts, and deaths: A meta-analysis and systematic review. *Journal of Psychiatric Research, 155*, 579–588. https://doi.org/10.1016/j.jpsychires.2022.09.050

Lester, D. (2000). The end of suicidology. *Crisis, 21*(4), 158–159. https://doi.org/10.1027/0227-5910.21.4.158

Li, X., Mu, F., Liu, D., Zhu, J., Yue, S., Liu, M., Liu, Y., & Wang, J. (2022). Predictors of suicidal ideation, suicide attempt and suicide death among people with major depressive disorder: A systematic review and meta-analysis of cohort studies. *Journal of Affective Disorders, 302*, 332–351. https://doi.org/10.1016/j.jad.2022.01.103

Macintyre, V. G., Mansell, W., Pratt, D., & Tai, S. J. (2021). The psychological pathway to suicide attempts: A strategy of control without awareness. *Frontiers in Psychology, 12*, 588683. https://doi.org/10.3389/fpsyg.2021.588683

Mann, J. J. (2003). Neurobiology of suicidal behaviour. *Nature Reviews. Neuroscience, 4*(10), 819–828. https://doi.org/10.1038/nrn1220

Mann, J. J., & Rizk, M. M. (2020). A brain-centric model of suicidal behavior. *The American Journal of Psychiatry, 177*(10), 902–916. https://doi.org/10.1176/appi.ajp.2020.20081224

Maung, H. H. (2020). Pluralism and incommensurability in suicide research. *Studies in History and Philosophy of Biological and Biomedical Sciences, 80*, 101247. https://doi.org/10.1016/j.shpsc.2019.101247

O'Connor, R. (2011). Towards an integrated motivational-volitional model of suicidal behaviour. In R. O'Connor, S. Platt, & J. Gordon (Eds.), *International handbook of suicide prevention: Research, policy, and practice* (pp. 181–198). Wiley-Blackwell.

O'Connor, R. C., & Kirtley, O. J. (2018). The integrated motivational-volitional model of suicidal behaviour. *Philosophical Transactions of the Royal Society of London. Series B, Biological Sciences, 373*(1754), 20170268. https://doi.org/10.1098/rstb.2017.0268

O'Connor, R. C., & Nock, M. K. (2014). The psychology of suicidal behaviour. *The Lancet. Psychiatry, 1*(1), 73–85. https://doi.org/10.1016/S2215-0366(14)70222-6

O'Connor, R. C., & Portzky, G. (2018). Looking to the future: A synthesis of new developments and challenges in suicide research and prevention. *Frontiers in Psychology, 9*, 2139. https://doi.org/10.3389/fpsyg.2018.02139

Rudd, M. (2006). Fluid vulnerability theory: A cognitive approach to understanding the process of acute and chronic suicide risk. In T. E. Ellis (Ed.), *Cognition and suicide: Theory, research, and therapy* (pp. 355–368). American Psychological Association.

Runeson, B., Odeberg, J., Pettersson, A., Edbom, T., Jildevik Adamsson, I., & Waern, M. (2017). Instruments for the assessment of suicide risk: A systematic review evaluating the certainty of the evidence. *PLoS One, 12*(7), e0180292. https://doi.org/10.1371/journal.pone.0180292

Schuck, A., Calati, R., Barzilay, S., Bloch-Elkouby, S., & Galynker, I. (2019). Suicide crisis syndrome: A review of supporting evidence for a new suicide-specific diagnosis. *Behavioral Sciences & the Law, 37*(3), 223–239. https://doi.org/10.1002/bsl.2397

Shneidman, E. S. (1993). *Suicide as psychache: A clinical approach to self-destructive behavior*. Jason Aronson.

Shneidman, E. S. (1998). Perspectives on suicidology. Further reflections on suicide and psychache. *Suicide & Life-Threatening Behavior, 28*(3), 245–250.

Stuckler, D., & Basu, S. (2013). *The body economic: Why austerity kills*. Basic Books.

Turecki, G., & Brent, D. A. (2016). Suicide and suicidal behaviour. *Lancet (London, England), 387*(10024), 1227–1239. https://doi.org/10.1016/S0140-6736(15)00234-2

Van Orden, K. A., Witte, T. K., Cukrowicz, K. C., Braithwaite, S. R., Selby, E. A., & Joiner, T. E., Jr. (2010). The interpersonal theory of suicide. *Psychological Review, 117*(2), 575–600. https://doi.org/10.1037/a0018697

van Rooij, I., & Baggio, G. (2020). Theory development requires an epistemological sea change. *Psychological Inquiry, 31*(4), 321–325. https://doi.org/10.1080/1047840X.2020.1853477

Wenzel, A., Brown, G. K., & Beck, A. T. (2009). *Cognitive therapy for suicidal patients: Scientific and clinical applications*. American Psychological Association.

White, J., Kral, M., Morris, J., & Marsh, I. (Eds.). (2016). *Critical suicidology: Transforming suicide research and prevention for the 21st century*. UBC Press.

Wray, M., Colen, C., & Pescosolido, B. (2011). The sociology of suicide. *Annual Review of Sociology, 37*, 505–528. https://doi.org/10.1146/annurev-soc-081309-150058

Young, J., Bishop, S., Humphrey, C., & Pavlacic, J. (2023). A review of natural language processing in the identification of suicidal behavior. *Journal of Affective Disorders Reports, 12*, 100507. https://doi.org/10.1016/j.jadr.2023.100507

Zortea, T. C., Cleare, S., Melson, A. J., Wetherall, K., & O'Connor, R. C. (2020). Understanding and managing suicide risk. *British Medical Bulletin, 134*(1), 73–84. https://doi.org/10.1093/bmb/ldaa013

Chapter 3
On the Psychodynamics of Suicidal Behaviors

Rui C. Campos

3.1 The Complex Nature of Suicidality

Human beings are aware of their own death and mortality, facilitated by their ability to construct representations and conceptualize death. This capacity enables individuals to contemplate and, in some cases, to take their own lives. Indeed, evolutionary perspectives suggest that humans are unique among animals in their capability to engage in self-destructive behavior. For example, Soper and Shackelford (2018) argued that: "An evolutionary analysis suggests that selection is unlikely to have tolerated the capacity for intentional self-killing in nonhuman animals. The potential to escape pain by suicide would have presented a recurrent and severe adaptive problem for an animal with a reproductive future to protect. If the potential for suicide arose in the evolutionary past, antisuicide mechanisms may have co-evolved, as we believe they have in adult humans" (Soper & Shackelford, 2018, p. 1). In other words, suicide in humans relates to "brain and pain."

It is usually accepted that suicidal behaviors represent a complex and multifaceted clinical phenomenon with causal factors that do not follow a linear trajectory. Currently, various explanatory psychological models have contributed to the current understanding of the suicidal process, each highlighting different specific factors associated with the emergence of suicidal ideation and behavior (Overholser et al., 2012). For example, three recent theories (the interpersonal theory of suicide, the integrated motivational-volitional model, and the three-step theory) have garnered considerable attention in contemporary research (O'Connor & Nock, 2014). These perspectives are framed within the framework of the transition from ideation to action and emphasize that the factors associated with suicidal ideation are distinct

R. C. Campos (✉)
Department of Psychology, School of Social Sciences and Comprehensive Health Research Centre, Universidade de Évora, Évora, Portugal
e-mail: rcampos@uevora.pt

Á. Jiménez-Molina, V. Martínez (eds.), *New Perspectives on Suicidal Behavior, Depression and Personality*, https://doi.org/10.1007/978-3-031-96037-6_3

from those subsequent influencing behavior, namely, suicide attempts or suicide (Klonsky & May, 2015; O'Connor & Nock, 2014).

Suicidal behaviors arise from a complex interplay of external and internal factors. Given that suicide and suicide attempts are complex phenomena, it is essential to adopt a modern perspective in psychopathology that recognizes *equifinality* (Cicchetti, 1990), meaning that different causes or factors can lead to the same outcome, such as psychopathological symptoms or suicidal behaviors, via different developmental pathways. Additionally, these behaviors may be associated with various factors in different individuals or at different stages of life.

Acknowledging the complex nature of suicidality, this chapter adopts a humanistic perspective on psychological pain and suffering. It focuses on the individual and their psychological functioning through a psychodynamic approach to explore the manifestations and experiences of (intolerable) suffering. This chapter provides a specific clinical perspective on the psychodynamics of suicidal behaviors, highlighting different elements related to depressive personality. Among other dimensions, it explores object relations linked to feelings of rejection and guilt, hopelessness and low self-esteem, a masochistic inner dimension and the need for atonement, anger directed toward the object that flows back on the self, a profound sense of disconnection, and a basic feeling of dissatisfaction, as well as the impulsivity and the "acting out" as mechanisms to deny or handle psychological suffering. Additionally, it briefly addresses the psychotherapeutic process and its ability to transform maladaptive objects and self-representations, thus fostering psychological growth and development.

3.2 From Psychache to the Psychological Meaning of Suicide

3.2.1 Psychache and Suicidal Behaviors

One of the central ideas of modern suicidology is that suicidal behavior is an act performed to stop intolerable psychological suffering. Shneidman (1993), the great suicidologist, wrote about 30 years ago an opening sentence that expresses an idea that has marked modern suicidology: "No psychache, no suicide" (p. 47). Despite psychache sharing some points with other inner aversive states, it is a unique entity (Orbach et al., 2003; Shneidman, 1993), theoretically and empirically distinct from other constructs such as distress, depression, or hopelessness (Campos et al., 2016; Campos & Holden, 2016; Troister & Holden, 2010, 2013). Psychache would result from the frustration of basic psychological needs (e.g., love and belonging, perceived control, positive self-image, meaningful relationships; Shneidman, 1990, 1998, 2005). However, psychache has different degrees, and suicide may only occur when its intensity crosses a threshold that shifts it to a unique qualitative state: when it is considered by the person to be unbearable (Shneidman, 1998). Psychological pain is an unavoidable concept when one intends to understand suicidal behaviors.

This theoretical conceptualization and the empirical results that other variables usually considered important, such as clinical depression, are linked to suicide risk through psychache (e.g., Campos et al., 2018; Campos & Holden, 2016) through a mediation effect, give us the ballast to think.

Several empirical studies attested to the importance of psychological pain in suicidality. For example, Campos et al. (2016) demonstrated, using data collected at two different time points, that psychache fully mediated the relationship between depressive symptoms and lifetime suicidality. In a longitudinal study, Spínola et al. (2022) demonstrated that changes over 5 months in psychache tended to mediate the relationship between childhood trauma and changes in suicidal ideation, controlling for depressive symptoms and thwarted interpersonal needs. Holden et al. (2020), with a convenience sample of 207 community adults and using logistic regression analysis, demonstrated that psychological pain provided a significant contribution in predicting lifetime self-harming behaviors, controlling for the significant co-variables of drug use and having a psychiatric diagnosis. In this same study, psychological pain also correlated with the frequency of lifetime self-harming behaviors, controlling for significant co-variables. Campos and Holden (2020), using two large samples of community adults and college students and logistic regression analyses, verified that psychache predicted lifetime suicide attempts for both samples, and Martins et al. (2022) with a sample of adults with a substance use disorder, and using path analysis by structural equation modeling found that depressive symptoms and low levels of managing psychological pain fully mediated the association between childhood trauma and suicidal ideation.

3.2.2 Psychodynamic Perspectives and the Psychological Meaning of Suicide

A more profound understanding of suicidal behaviors requires taking a look at their psychological meanings. Is the human being able to dispose of his/her life also as a way of denying or controlling the anguish of death? It is conceivable that certain risk-taking behaviors serve as attempts to deny or mitigate this anguish of death. Consider, for instance, the image of a teenager astride a motorcycle, navigating a bustling thoroughfare with reckless abandon—speeding, weaving through traffic, heedless of the perilous consequences. At this moment, there seems to be a willful blindness to inherent mortality, an inability or unwillingness to acknowledge the real potential for self-destruction. On the one hand, the image evokes Baechler's (1975) concept of "playful suicide," which he defined as a way of engaging or playing with life. Baechler defined different types of suicide, but all constitute a form of behavior that seeks a solution to an existential crisis. On the other hand, this image suggests the absence of fear of physical pain and death as an indispensable dimension for suicidal behavior (Joiner, 2005).

In psychodynamic psychology and psychopathology, explaining inherently involves understanding, leading us to consider the concept of psychological meaning. What, then, might be the psychological significance of suicidal behavior as a risk-taking action? The psychological "function" of such behavior may vary depending on the individual's age or stage in the life cycle. In adolescence, for example, suicidal behaviors may represent an attitude of defiance in the face of authority or may symbolize a desire for rebirth. Differently, in old age, suicide may express profound feelings of disconnection and loneliness or a desire for a reunion with already deceased relatives.

From a psychodynamic perspective, apart from serving as a paradoxical way of managing anxiety and anguish of death, risk behaviors can also reflect feelings of guilt and the need for atonement or expiation. Additionally, they may manifest as impulsive and aggressive movements directed towards significant others; suicide as a form of revenge, blackmail, or manipulation (Baechler, 1975).

Furthermore, suicidal behaviors and other risky behaviors may represent an attitude of defiance, a challenge to authority that is particularly evident in some teenage suicide attempts—a symbolic way to access power, to demonstrate control, at least over one's own body and one's own life. They can also function as a cry for help or a means of escape, allowing adolescents to distance themselves from relationships that cause emotional pain and distress. Ringel (1976), for example, observed that suicidal behaviors could be seen as a means of escaping an intolerable situation and as a desperate cry for help. Shneidman (1993) also considered that suicide often constitutes an attempt to seek relief when all other options seem unviable, with many suicidal acts being cries for help and a way to communicate profound psychological suffering. According to Grinberg (2000), unconscious fantasies that may contribute to suicide include the desire to escape reality or to enter a state akin to sleep—conceiving death as a form of eternal slumber.

Alternatively, suicide may symbolize a desire for rebirth or the desire to start a new life. For example, when communication with significant others fails, "the young person wants to kill himself but does not wish to die" but instead intends to metaphorically "be born again" (Sampaio, 1997, p. 401). This interpretation hints at the fantasy of reuniting or establishing a new relationship with the significant others.

From a psychodynamic perspective, suicidal behavior may also be associated with feelings of persecutory guilt deserving of punishment: "I am sorry, I have hurt everyone; they are better off without me" (Grinberg, 2000). Another fantasy involves a hostile desire for revenge and exerting control beyond death. In some cases, a consequence of this may be the guilt felt by survivors, believing that somehow they were responsible for the suicidal act. This guilt can partially explain an increased risk of suicide among survivors themselves.

Moreover, a desire for masochistic submission could lead to a state of ecstasy, serving as a means of reunion with the deceased loved one. Zibboorg (1936) emphasized an ethnocultural model of suicide and the identification of the individual with the deceased, which could culminate in suicide by reunion. This concept helps elucidate suicides that occur on specific dates, such as the anniversary of a deceased relative.

3.3 Depressive Personality and Suicidality

From a psychodynamic perspective, various elements of the psychological functioning can help to understand the suicidal act: object relations associated with feelings of rejection and guilt, a masochistic dimension and the need for atonement, a deficit in self-esteem (with feelings of unworthiness and smallness), and anger directed at the object that ultimately falls back on the Self. Additionally, significant factors include a profound sense of disconnection, fundamental dissatisfaction, hopelessness, and a decrease in libido (Campos, 2014, 2016); psychological pain, in a broad sense, as a pervasive factor associated with the intolerability of the person's situation. Moreover, impulsivity or "acting out" can be ways of denying, mitigating, or "managing" this profound suffering.

From this perspective, it is almost inevitable to situate suicidal behavior within the context of depressive psychological functioning. Depression, in a broad sense, is related to a lack of meaning in life and can create a situation of intolerable psychological pain. It is within the framework of this psychological pain and depressive functioning that the motivation for suicidal acts makes sense, rather than solely within the context of clinical depression in the psychiatric sense. While the significance and relative importance of different depressive personality traits can vary between individuals and within the same person over time, depressive functioning is generally characterized by a severe superego and a pervasive sense of guilt, often linked to a masochistic dimension of the personality. This state may also involve narcissistic injury, feelings of rejection, loneliness, and detachment, as well as a profound sense of dissatisfaction, hopelessness, and emptiness. Additionally, it is often accompanied by a decline in libidinal energy and self-directed anger.

3.3.1 Masochistic and Narcissistic Reasons for Suicide

As several psychoanalysts have described (e.g., Bowlby, 1969; Coimbra de Matos, 2001), depressive personality often originates from childhood experiences of affective rejection and loss, leading to a deficit in the narcissism. As a result of this narcissistic wound, individuals with a depressive personality tend to be particularly sensitive to various types of loss throughout their lives. However, because both loss and narcissistic vulnerability are challenging to accept, they are often denied.

Another key feature of the depressive personality is its masochistic dimension (Freud, 1917), which manifests in suffering as a means of seeking recognition—even beyond death. This perspective helps explaining the phenomenon in which some individuals experience a sense of relief or even well-being in the moments preceding a suicidal act. Furthermore, suicide can be understood as an attempt to transition toward something perceived as better than their current existence (Baechler, 1975).

Furthermore, many times, the experience during the individual's final moments is influenced by the psychotic part of the personality (Bion, 1962), which takes control and serves the will to die. In other words, a failure in reality testing and a regressive psychotic movement can be observed, explaining the "courage" to follow through with the suicidal act. This act is often perceived as heroic when, in reality, it reflects a psychotic regression—a moment of psychological breakdown or "madness" (Grinberg, 2000).

Another way to die heroically is to let oneself die or die slowly. This can manifest in a lack of self-care, subjecting oneself to multiple injuries or bodily harm, or the absence of healthy behaviors that, through cumulative effect, damage the body. It can also present as being the victim of a serious accident, which unconsciously represents a way of killing oneself. These cases can reveal the masochistic core of the depressive personality.

In some suicidal acts, the intention to die may be absent from consciousness, although the individual places themselves in situations where their behavior can lead to death (Sampaio, 1997). These different forms of risky behavior could be an expression of a "compulsion to repeat" (Freud, 1914), referring to a form of acting out and self-destructive intention. As it is well known, the compulsion to repeat refers to an unconscious tendency of an individual to repeat painful experiences, even if they are harmful to him/herself (Freud, 1920/2009). This compulsion can manifest when an individual continuously relives from traumatic feelings of despair, repeatedly engaging in self-destructive actions as an attempt to master or alleviate these unbearable emotional states.

In other cases, such as some suicides that occur in advanced ages, there may be an existential balance marked by failure and a harsh awareness of what the person could and wished to have done. Here, suicide may appear as an acceptable solution that interrupts an existence of suffering and failure, whether real or imagined, but intolerable. In other words, suicide alleviates the pain of a narcissistic wound (Coimbra de Matos, 2001).

All these cases refer to masochistic and narcissistic reasons for suicide, with the latter being associated with the inability to bear a wounded narcissism and the collapse of self-esteem. It is then a case of an "impossible mourning" or an "uncompleted mourning" (Coimbra de Matos, 1982), the mourning of a lost time or a lost object (Klein, 1952, 1957), an eternal mourning. There may be no greater longing for what was fervently desired in fantasy, in the inner world, but was never possible to achieve. Depression is composed of this nostalgia. This helps to understand the suicidal act as the result of a loss of the desire to live, not necessarily as a desire to die. From this perspective, it is also possible to understand depression as the disease of loss, the loss of something that one has never indeed had (for a development of this topic, see Leader, 2008).

3.3.2 Rejection and Suicidality

Is there a loss of the desire to live in suicide, or rather, a desire to live another life? Often, people who have attempted suicide express the desire to live a different life, a more dignified life. In many of these cases, especially among adolescents, the suicidal act can assume an appealing or communicative meaning, representing an attempt to escape from a profound sense of disconnection, loneliness, or lack of belonging. The lack of a sense of belonging may originate from rejection and be linked to identity diffusion. These two aspects—rejection and identity diffusion—are intimately connected, as we only indeed "exist" because we were loved: We only "exist" because we exist for someone (Campos, 2009).

On the other hand, the desire to live another life (not the desire to die) results from a profound dissatisfaction from not meeting the basic affective needs of the Self (Kohut, 1971). Besides other needs, the need for appreciation, belonging, acceptance, and identification with "good" objects are essential, and their profound frustration is associated with psychopathological manifestations such as depression.

Several studies have shown the importance of parental rejection in suicidal behavior. For example, Campos et al. (2013), using a sample of community adults and an analysis based on structural equation modeling (SEM), demonstrated that recollections of parental rejection had a significant direct association with suicidality and was significantly associated with self-criticism. That same self-criticism was significantly associated with depressive symptoms, which, in turn, were significantly associated with suicidality. Thus, the authors concluded that individuals who perceived more parental rejection were at greater risk of suicide ideation and behaviors, possibly because such experiences predispose them to intense self-criticism. Sobrinho et al. (2016), with a sample of young adults evaluated at two different times points observed that parental rejection was directly and indirectly related to suicidality, mediated by self-criticism and depressive symptoms.

It is also known that individuals with a depressive personalitiy tend to idealize significant others who seem to have fallen short of their desire (Coimbra de Matos, 2001). However, the actual negative characteristics of these objects are denied or repressed, as the child cannot survive without these relationships. In some cases, however, during adolescence or adulthood, the actual characteristics of the objects are no longer denied, and a harsh conscience emerges as an unbearable burden: "I was not accepted and loved as I am!". From this perspective, suicidal behaviors can be interpreted, at least partially, as the realization of a particular infanticidal desire. The anger toward the object is actually directed against the Self, which identifies with the object (Freud, 1917). However, this "anti-depressive" mechanism generates a disruption in the Self that is invaded by the aggressiveness of the object.

3.3.3 A Demanding Superego and Self-Criticism

An important aspect of psychodynamic theory regarding suicidal behavior centers on a demanding superego that generates feelings of unworthiness and guilt. This guilt intensifies masochism and can contribute to the suicidal act, giving it a meaning of atonement but also of liberation. Menninger (1938) argued that every person at suicidal risk has three desires: to kill, to be killed, and to die. A destructive impulse characterizes the first desire, while the second desire, to be killed, stems from guilt and the need to be punished by the superego. The third desire expresses the longing to return to the maternal womb (Menninger, 1938).

Similarly, Grinberg (2000) states that individuals may resort to suicide as the only escape from persecutory guilt directed at themselves by a severe and overwhelming superego. One of the fantasies of the person attempting suicide, of an omnipotent/magical nature, is that through suicide, he/she can direct aggression against their internal persecutors, thereby getting rid of them. In this way, death is experienced as a release from these internal persecutory objects. Additionally, a manic defense of denial of one's own death may play a role in this dynamic. According to Grinberg, the central core of suicidal behaviors always revolves around persecutory guilt. Sometimes, the person at suicidal risk projects this unbearable guilt onto others, experiencing this projection as a triumph over them: "I kill myself so that you bear the guilt."

A similar dynamic can be observed in cases of suicidal behaviors in children. In these cases, self-destruction can represent punishment by the superego due to the child's identification with their parents, who are generally very severe and demanding. Sometimes, there is even a conscious attitude on the part of the child to punish the parents for their hostility, or rather, a desire to reunite through death with images of good or idealized objects (Grinberg, 2000).

In the context of clinical research, it has been observed that ruminations on self-worth, self-esteem, failure, and guilt can be particularly insidious in individuals with an introjective depressive personality (Blatt, 2004, 2008), making them vulnerable to serious suicide attempts. Clinical reports and media references have illustrated the suicidal potential of highly talented, ambitious, and successful individuals who are nonetheless plagued by intense, painful introspection, self-doubt, guilt, and self-criticism. Blatt (1995, 2004) described an introspective/self-critical vulnerability to depression characterized by feelings of unworthiness, inferiority, guilt, and failure. Vulnerable individuals engage in rigorous self-evaluation and have a chronic fear of criticism. They strive hard for success and perfection, are often highly competitive, and work tirelessly, placing many demands on themselves and often achieving significant results, but with only short-lived feelings of satisfaction. Due to their intense competitiveness, they can be critical and aggressive towards others. Through overcompensation mechanisms, they strive to achieve and maintain approval and recognition.

Various studies indicate that self-critical vulnerability plays an important role in suicidal ideation and behavior and is closely related to the lethality of suicidal behaviors (Fazaa & Page, 2003; Morrison & O'Connor, 2007; O'Connor, 2007). For example, Fazaa and Page (2003) found that introjective/self-critical college students who attempted suicide had a greater intent to die and made more serious attempts than anaclitic/dependent suicidal students. In another study, Campos et al. (2012) found that the introjective/self-critical personality style was related to suicidality in a sample of community adults. However, this relationship was mediated by depression, hostility, anxiety, and interpersonal sensitivity. In a longitudinal study with a community sample, Campos et al. (2018) demonstrated that changes in self-criticism predicted changes in suicidal ideation after statistically controlling for changes in distress. Changes in the interaction between self-criticism and distress predicted changes in suicidal ideation. Campos and Holden (2016) tested a comprehensive mediation model, including maladaptive traits of self-criticism and neediness as exogenous variables, with depressive symptoms, psychache, and thwarted interpersonal needs as mediators. The results of this study show that self-criticism and neediness were related to depression, which in turn was related to suicidality through psychache and thwarted interpersonal needs.

3.3.4 Anger Against Self and Decrease in Inner Energy

According to Freud (1917), in melancholia, self-destructive behavior involved a sadistic superego attacking a fragile and masochistic ego. Following the identification with the ambivalent object, the aggression that has been introjected, the anger against the object falls back on the Self. The clinical observation that anger directed at the Self is a hallmark of depressive personality and is linked to suicide risk has been supported by empirical research. For example, Campos et al. (2011) tested the relationship between defense mechanisms according to Ihilevich and Gleser's perspective (1986, 1991) and the maladaptive depressive traits of neediness and self-criticism. According to the results, Turning Against Self was related to both types of maladaptive depressive traits.

Freud (1920) developed the idea of the "death drive" when he observed the brutality of the First World War. However, is there an excess of the death drive in suicidal behavior? Or should the question be posed differently? Is it possible to consider the presence of a death-object relationship?

From a classic psychoanalytic perspective, the death drive and its derivatives constitute one of the specific aspects that would determine the human vulnerability to suicide (Litman, 1966). Nevertheless, does the person at suicidal risk truly desire death or simply does not desire life? In most people, the desire to live predominates over the desire to die. It is precisely this ambivalence that makes suicide prevention possible (Grinberg, 2000).

Anyway, there is a presence of death in life; death haunts life: some deny it, others challenge it, and still others study and think about it. But at the same time, there can often be "life" in suicidal behavior, a desire to live. There is a massive decrease in desire/energy in the person at suicidal risk when considering suicide in light of depressive personality functioning. However, even so, there is psychological energy available to take one's own life, to be able to end life, even momentarily. From where does this energy come from? Clinical work allows one to think that an object may become autonomous within the person; an introjection of malignancy/aggressiveness. This malign object may have a very particular "triple structure": a fragile, absent, and alienating part; another persecutory, envious, and invasive part; and yet another, deeply depressed, incapable of mourning the ideal child: "You are not as I wanted, so I cannot accept you as you are!" (Campos, 2018).

It could be argued that some individuals die prematurely due to nonreciprocity, a lack of belonging—feeling as though they have no right to exist—and the absence of a meaningful connection with others and, most importantly, with themselves.

3.4 A Brief Reference to the Psychoanalytic Psychotherapeutic Process

The dimensions and mechanisms mentioned above, from a psychodynamic perspective, highlight the challenge involved in clinical work with individuals at risk of suicide. The affectionate gaze of an attentive, unconcerned but interested other, akin to a mirror and the maternal face of that good initial mother who perhaps was not truly there, can help to glimpse a way out and promote understanding, elaboration, acceptance, and psychological growth in people at risk for suicide (Campos, 2017). It has likely never been more important to give voice to the individual, their inner world, and their existence. Psychodynamic psychotherapy aims to analyze and "repair" the past while strengthening the individual's identity and establishing significant bonds with others. This process allows the individual to look to the future with greater hope. In psychotherapy, as in the developmental process, psychological growth and development occur through a combination of moments of connection and separation, of involvement and incompatibility (Blatt et al., 2008).

Internalization throughout the therapeutic process occurs similarly to normative development: through a progressive spiral of gratifying involvement with objects and experiences of incompatibility, approximation, and moments of separation in a unique relationship (Blatt et al., 2008). This dialectical interaction allows for an evolution towards more mature forms of interpersonal relationships and a more integrated and differentiated sense of the Self. A parallel between the psychotherapeutic process and childhood experience is the possibility and the need for the client to be recognized as possessing subjectivity, mental capacity, and individuality. In this line, Fonagy and Target (2005) highlight the importance of the patient experiencing that the psychotherapist can develop a coherent model of two minds meeting: *trought the experience of a mind's having their minds in mind*. From the perspective of intersubjectivity, this also allows the patient to recognize the therapist's subjectivity and independence. The ability to observe and understand the Self and others constitutes a meta-capacity of mentalization that several authors consider an essential factor for change in psychotherapy (Fonagy & Target, 2005).

The activation of distorted representations of significant objects in the therapeutic process provides the patient and therapist with the opportunity to observe, understand, and review these representations, which may be hostile, critical, demanding, sadistic, and complementary to a representation of the Self as unworthy, alone, suffering, annulled, and diminished. This review allows for constructing new schemas (Blatt & Luyten, 2009). The new internalizations are expressed behaviorally and psychologically in more mature levels of identity and relationships with others, in the development of new adaptive abilities, in a greater understanding of the Self and others (Blatt et al., 2010), in the reduction of symptoms and risky behaviors, and a greater joy for life, making death no longer seem like an option or solution.

3.5 Final Words

One day, a student asked me why I was interested in studying suicidal behaviors. I remained silent for a moment; I had not thought it much before. However, at that moment, something occurred to me: to study suicidality—the motivation to die—is, in a way, to seek meaning in life. It is also an act of celebrating life. May we always find ways to celebrate life, even when pain overwhelms us. May we never lose the ability to dream. Mia Couto, a writer from Mozambique, a Portuguese-speaking country in Africa, captures this idea beautifully in one of his books:

> “"Does it hurt you anything?";
> “It is the life that hurts, doctor.”
> “And what do you do when the pain strikes?”
> “What I do best, Your Excellency.”
> “And what is that?”
> “I dream.”

It seems fitting to conclude by emphasizing that, in both the beginning and the end, what matters most is human connection. I recall the words of a renowned Portuguese suicidologist Daniel Sampaio: “Even when one dies, one does not die alone.” Allow me to put it another way: When you die, you die alone—always alone. However, even in death, no one truly wishes to be alone.

References

Baechler, J. (1975). *Les suicides*. Alcan.

Bion, W. R. (1962). A theory of thinking. *International Journal of Psychoanalysis, 43*, 306–310.

Blatt, S. J. (1995). The destructiveness of perfectionism. Implications for the treatment of depression. *The American Psychologist, 50*(12), 1003–1020. https://doi.org/10.1037/0003-066x.50.12.1003

Blatt, S. J. (2004). *Experiences of depression: Theoretical, research and clinical perspectives*. American Psychological Association.
Blatt, S. J. (2008). *Polarities of experience: Relatedness and self-definition in personality development, psychopathology, and the therapeutic process*. American Psychological Association.
Blatt, S. J., Auerbach, J. S., & Behrends, R. S. (2008). Changes in the representation of self and significant others in the treatment process: Links between representation, internalization, and mentalization. In E. L. Jurist, A. Slade, & S. Bergner (Eds.), *Mind to mind: Infant research, neuroscience, and psychoanalysis* (pp. 225–263). Other Press.
Blatt, S. J., & Luyten, P. (2009). A structural-developmental psychodynamic approach to psychopathology: Two polarities of experience across the life span. *Development and Psychopathology, 21*(3), 793–814. https://doi.org/10.1017/S0954579409000431
Blatt, S. J., Zuroff, D. C., Hawley, L. L., & Auerbach, J. S. (2010). Predictors of sustained therapeutic change. *Psychotherapy Research, 20*(1), 37–54. https://doi.org/10.1080/10503300903121080
Bowlby, J. (1969). *Attachment and loss*. Basic Books.
Campos, R. C. (2009). E quando o corpo fala…: Expressões somáticas da psicopatologia. *Saúde Mental, 11*, 42–47. [When the body speaks: Somatic expressions of psychopathology].
Campos, R. C. (2014). Porque não posso viver assim, aceito antes de tempo o meu fim: Uma reflexão sobre suicídio. *Revista Portuguesa de Psicanálise e Psicoterapia Psicanalítica, 5*, 97–118. [Because I can not live like this I acccpt my carly cnd: Thinking about suicide].
Campos, R. C. (2016). Dor psíquica e risco de suicídio. Notas para uma compreensão dos comportamentos suicidários. *Revista Portuguesa de Psicanálise e Psicoterapia Psicanalítica, 7*, 103–112. [Mental pain and suicide risk: Notes for a comprehension of suicidal behaviours.].
Campos, R. C. (2017) *Dor psíquica, intolerabilidade e suicídio: Notas para um entendimento psicanalítico dos comportamentos suicidários*. Conferência, no âmbito da formação de psicoterapeutas na PsiRelacional—Associação de Psicanálise Relacional. Lisboa 17 de Fevereiro. [Psychological pain, intolerability and suicide: Notes to a psychoanalytic understanding of suicidal behaviours].
Campos, R. C. (2018). Será que o amor pode matar? Um olhar psicanalítico sobre o amor, a morte e o suicídio. Comunicação apresentada no colóquio *Psicanálise para o século XXI*. Lisboa, 26 e 27 de Outubro. [Can love kill: A psychoanalytic approach of love, death and suicide].
Campos, R. C., Besser, A., & Blatt, S. J. (2011). The relationships between defenses and experiences of depression: An exploratory study. *Psychoanalytic Psychology, 28*(2), 196–208. https://doi.org/10.1037/a0022420
Campos, R. C., Besser, A., & Blatt, S. J. (2012). Distress mediates the association between personality predispositions and suicidality: A preliminary study in a Portuguese community sample. *Archives of Suicide Research, 16*(1), 44–58. https://doi.org/10.1080/13811118.2012.640583
Campos, R. C., Besser, A., & Blatt, S. J. (2013). Recollections of parental rejection, self-criticism and depression in suicidality. *Archives of Suicide Research, 17*(1), 58–74. https://doi.org/10.1080/13811118.2013.748416
Campos, R. C., & Holden, R. R. (2016). Testing a theory-based model of suicidality in a community sample. *Omega: Journal of Death and Dying, 74*(2), 119–137. https://doi.org/10.1177/0030222815598428
Campos, R. C., & Holden, R. R. (2020). Psychological pain and previous suicide attempts in young adults: Results with the Portuguese version of the Psychache Scale. *Journal of Clinical Psychology, 76*(10), 1965–1971. https://doi.org/10.1002/jclp.22973
Campos, R. C., Holden, R. R., Baleizão, C., Caçador, B., & Fragata, A. S. (2018). Self-criticism, neediness, and distress in the prediction of suicide ideation: Results from cross-sectional and longitudinal studies. *The Journal of Psychology, 152*(4), 237–255. https://doi.org/10.1080/00223980.2018.1446895
Campos, R. C., Holden, R. R., Laranjeira, P., Troister, T., Oliveira, A. R., Costa, F., Abreu, M., & Fresca, N. (2016). Self-report depressive symptoms do not directly predict suicidality in nonclinical individuals: Contributions toward a more psychosocial approach to suicide risk. *Death Studies, 40*(6), 335–349. https://doi.org/10.1080/07481187.2016.1150920

Cicchetti, D. (1990). A historical perspective on the discipline of developmental psychopathology. In J. Rolf & A. S. Masten (Eds.), *Risk and protective factors in the development of psychopathology*. Cambridge University Press.

Coimbra de Matos, A. (1982). Razões da more, morte da razão: Abordagem psicanalítica do suicídio. *Conferências apresentada no Encontro: "A morte vista por"*, Lisboa, 28 a 29 de Janeiro. [Reasons of death, death of reason: A psychoanalytic approach to suicide].

Coimbra de Matos, A. (2001). *Depressão. Episódios de um percurso em busca do seu sentido*. Climepsi. [Depression. Episodes from a journey in search of meaning].

Fazaa, N., & Page, S. (2003). Dependency and self-criticism as predictors of suicidal behavior. *Suicide & Life-Threatening Behavior, 33*(2), 172–185. https://doi.org/10.1521/suli.33.2.172.22777

Fonagy, P., & Target, M. (2005). Some reflections on the therapeutic action of psychoanalytic therapy. In J. S. Auerbach, K. N. Levy, & C. E. Schaffer (Eds.), *Relatedness, self-definition, and mental representation: Essays in honor of Sidney J. Blatt* (pp. 191–212). Routledge.

Freud, S. (1914). Remembering, repeating and working-throug. The Standard Edition of the Complete Psychological Works of Sigmund Freud.

Freud, S. (1917). Mourning and melancholia. The Standard Edition of the Complete Psychological Works of Sigmund Freud.

Freud, S. (1920/2009). Para além do princípio do prazer. Relogio D'Agua. [Beyond the pleasure principle].

Grinberg, L. (2000). *Culpa e depressão*. Climepsi. [Guilt and depression].

Holden, R. R., Campos, R. C., & Lambert, C. E. (2020). Psychological pain and self-harming behaviours in an adulthood community sample: An exploratory study. *European Journal of Psychiatry, 34*, 173–176. https://doi.org/10.1016/j.ejpsy.2020.03.001

Ihilevich, D., & Gleser, G. C. (1986). *Defense mechanisms: Their classification, correlates, and measurement with the defense mechanisms inventory*. DMI Associates.

Ihilevich, D., & Gleser, G. C. (1991). *Defenses in psychotherapy: The clinical application of the defense mechanisms inventory*. DMI Associates.

Joiner, T. (2005). *Why people die by suicide*. Harvard University Press.

Klein, M. (1952/1991). Algumas conclusões teóricas relativas à vida emocional do bebê. *Obras Completas de Melanie Klein (Volume III) Inveja e Gratidão e outros trabalhos*. Imago. [Some theoretical conclusions about the emotional life of the infant].

Klein, M. (1957/1991). Inveja e Gratidão. Obras Completas de Melanie Klein (Volume III) Inveja e Gratidão e outros trabalhos. Imago. [Envy and gratitude].

Klonsky, E. D., & May, A. M. (2015). The three-step theory (3ST): A new theory of suicide rooted in the "ideation-to-action" framework. *International Journal of Cognitive Therapy, 8*(2), 114–129. https://doi.org/10.1521/ijct.2015.8.2.114

Kohut, H. (1971). *The analysis of the self*. International University Press.

Leader, D. (2008). *The new black: Mourning, melancholia, and depression*. Graywolf Press.

Litman, R. E. (1966). Sigmund Freud on suicide. *The Psychoanalytic Forum, 1*, 206–214.

Martins, L. C., Campos, R. C., & Morujão, I. S. (2022). The mediating role of tolerance for psychological pain in the relationship of childhood trauma to suicidal ideation in individuals with a substance use disorder. *The British Journal of Clinical Psychology, 61*(2), 197–213. https://doi.org/10.1111/bjc.12338

Menninger, K. (1938). *Man against himself*. Harcourt.

Morrison, R., & O'Connor, R. C. (2007). *Suicidal thinking and psychological distress: The role of ruminative response style*. Presented at the XXIV World Congress of the International Association for Suicide Prevention, Killarney, Ireland.

O'Connor, R. C. (2007). The relations between perfectionism and suicidality: A systematic review. *Suicide & Life-Threatening Behavior, 37*(6), 698–714. https://doi.org/10.1521/suli.2007.37.6.698

O'Connor, R. C., & Nock, M. K. (2014). The psychology of suicidal behaviour. *The lancet. Psychiatry, 1*(1), 73–85. https://doi.org/10.1016/S2215-0366(14)70222-6

Orbach, I., Mikulincer, M., Gilboa-Schechtman, E., & Sirota, P. (2003). Mental pain and its relationship to suicidality and life meaning. *Suicide & Life-Threatening Behavior, 33*(3), 231–241. https://doi.org/10.1521/suli.33.3.231.23213

Overholser, J. C., Braden, A., & Dieter, L. (2012). Understanding suicide risk: Identification of high-risk groups during high-risk times. *Journal of Clinical Psychology, 68*(3), 349–361. https://doi.org/10.1002/jclp.20859

Ringel, E. (1976). The presuicidal syndrome. *Suicide & Life-Threatening Behavior, 6*(3), 131–149.

Sampaio, D. (1997). Suicido e parasuicidio. In J. C. Dias Cordeiro (Ed.), Manual de psiquiatria clínica (pp 395–403). Fundação Calouste Gulbenkian

Shneidman, E. S. (1990). The commonalities of suicide across the life span. In A. A. Leenaars (Ed.), *Life span perspectives of suicide*. Springer. https://doi.org/10.1007/978-1-4899-0724-0_4

Shneidman, E. S. (1993). Suicide as psychache. *The Journal of Nervous and Mental Disease, 181*(3), 145–147. https://doi.org/10.1097/00005053-199303000-00001

Shneidman, E. S. (1998). Perspectives on suicidology. Further reflections on suicide and psychache. *Suicide & Life-Threatening Behavior, 28*(3), 245–250.

Shneidman, E. S. (2005). Anodyne psychotherapy for suicide: A psychological view of suicide. *Clinical Neuropsychiatry: Journal of Treatment Evaluation, 2*(1), 7–12.

Sobrinho, A. T., Campos, R. C., & Holden, R. R. (2016). Parental rejection, personality, and depression in the prediction of suicidality in a sample of nonclinical young adults. *Psychoanalytic Psychology, 33*(4), 554–570. https://doi.org/10.1037/pap0000051

Soper, C. A., & Shackelford, T. K. (2018). If nonhuman animals can suicide, why don't they? *Animal Sentience, 2*(20), 14.

Spínola, J., Campos, R. C., Marques, D., & Holden, R. R. (2022). Psychache, unmet interpersonal needs, childhood trauma and suicide ideation in young adults. *Death Studies, 46*(4), 930–939. https://doi.org/10.1080/07481187.2020.1788670

Troister, T., & Holden, R. R. (2010). Comparing psychache, depression, and hopelessness in their associations with suicidality: A test of Shneidman's theory of suicide. *Personality and Individual Differences, 49*, 689–693. https://doi.org/10.1016/j.paid.2010.06.006

Troister, T., & Holden, R. R. (2013). Factorial differentiation among depression, hopelessness, and psychache in statistically predicting suicidality. *Measurement and Evaluation in Counseling and Development, 46*(1), 50–63. https://doi.org/10.1177/0748175612451744

Zibboorg, G. (1936). Differential diagnostic types of suicide. *Archives of Neurology and Psychiatry, 35*, 270–291.

Chapter 4
Reexamining the Role of Suicidal Behavior in Personality Disorder: Current Diagnostic Considerations and Cultural Variability

Alex Behn and Carla Sharp

4.1 Behavioral Dysregulation, Suicidal Behavior, and Personality Disorders

Most mental health clinicians would readily recognize the spectra of behavioral dysregulation as a typical component of the diagnosis of a personality disorder. Behavioral dysregulation is a multifaceted construct that includes general impulsive or reckless behavior, aggressive behaviors, suicidal ideation and suicide attempts, and non-suicidal self-injury (NSSI). In this regard, behavioral dysregulation can be conceptualized as a transdiagnostic precursor of suicidal behavior (Benton et al., 2021). Behavioral dysregulation, however, is also considered to be a transdiagnostic phenomenon, underlying many psychopathological presentations as severity increases. Thus, it is of interest to examine what might be transdiagnostic and what might be specific about behavioral dysregulation and specifically about suicidal behavior in personality disorders.

The diagnosis of personality disorders has evolved from a categorical approach in which ten personality disorders are viewed as discret, delimited entities to, more recently, a dimensional approach, culminating in the DSM-5's Alternative Model for Personality Disorders (AMPD), which integrates both categorical and dimensional diagnostic criteria (Sharp & Wall, 2021). From this new perspective, a personality disorder is a type of mental disorder characterized by enduring patterns of maladaptive self- and interpersonal functioning (Krueger & Hobbs, 2020).

A. Behn (✉)
School of Psychology, Pontificia Universidad Católica de Chile, Santiago, Chile

Millennium Institute for Research in Depression and Personality (MIDAP), Santiago, Chile
e-mail: albehn@uc.cl

C. Sharp
Department of Psychology, University of Houston, Houston, TX, USA

Á. Jiménez-Molina, V. Martínez (eds.), *New Perspectives on Suicidal Behavior*, Depression and Personality, https://doi.org/10.1007/978-3-031-96037-6_4

According to the AMPD in the DSM-5, personality disorders are defined by two primary criteria: Criterion A, which involves the severity of impaired personality functioning (self- and interpersonal functioning), and Criterion B, which involves specific maladaptive personality traits.

Personality disorders are relatively stable over time, begin in adolescence or early adulthood, and cause significant distress or impairment in social, occupational, or other important areas of functioning. The diagnosis and understanding of personality disorders emphasize individuals' dynamic and subjective experiences, reflecting the complexities of human behavior and personality, including the subjective experience of the self (Sharp & Wall, 2021). Suicidal behavior is significantly increased in the presence of a mental disorder (Arsenault-Lapierre et al., 2004), and a specific diagnosis of personality disorder further elevates the probability of a repeated attempt (de la Torre et al., 2023). Suicidal behavior in personality disorders represents a significant concern due to the high prevalence and severe impact of these disorders globally. According to a comprehensive meta-analysis, personality disorders affect approximately 7.8% of the global population, with higher rates observed in high-income countries compared to low- and middle-income countries (LMICs) (Winsper et al., 2020). This widespread prevalence underscores the critical need to address the mental health challenges associated with these disorders.

Furthermore, individuals with personality disorders exhibit substantially elevated risks of suicidal behavior and self-injury. Studies reveal that up to 80% of individuals diagnosed with borderline personality disorder (BPD) engage in NSSI, and a significant portion attempts suicide, with about 9% ultimately dying from suicide (McClelland et al., 2023). This highlights the urgent necessity for targeted interventions and comprehensive diagnostic considerations to mitigate the profound personal and societal costs associated with suicidal behaviors in personality disorders. The cultural variability in the expression and recognition of these disorders further complicates their diagnosis and treatment, necessitating culturally sensitive approaches to address this global mental health priority effectively.

4.1.1 Impulsivity and Reckless Behavior and Its Relationship with Negative Affect

Impulsivity and reckless behavior are transdiagnostic features present in a wide range of mental health disorders and problems, frequently termed impulsivity-related disorders (Valenciano-Mendoza et al., 2022). These disorders include, among others, addiction disorders, attention deficit hyperactivity disorder (ADHD), conduct disorder, bipolar disorder, eating disorders, obsessive-compulsive disorder, and personality disorders, mainly antisocial and borderline expressions of personality disorder (Pearlstein et al., 2024). However, it is not clear if manifestations of impulsivity across disorders express the same pathways and mechanisms. Even though transdiagnostic in nature, facets of impulsive behavior have been consistently related to personality disorder, specifically to the borderline and antisocial expression of personality disorder. Consistently, patients diagnosed with BPD will exhibit higher impulsivity traits than healthy controls (Sebastian et al., 2013). A review of impulsivity in personality disorder conducted by McHugh and Balaratnasingam (2018) concluded that problems in inhibitory control and discounting of rewards (i.e., a preference for smaller but immediate rewards) are both independently related to BPD and constitute stable features of the disorder. The spectrum of impulsivity also appears to be prominent in antisocial personality disorder (ASPD). In this case, the influence of emotional distress as a correlate of impulsive behavior does not appear to be quite as important as in the case of BPD (Turner et al., 2017). In general, facets of impulsive behavior may partially explain the frequent comorbidity of personality disorder with substance and alcohol use disorder (Koudys et al., 2023) and with attentional deficit disorder (Ditrich et al., 2021). Interestingly, cognitive functioning does not appear to be related to impulsivity in personality disorder. However, especially in BPD, impulsivity appears to be primarily present in the setting of intense negative emotions or increased distress (Turner et al., 2017). This finding supporting negative urgency as a model to examine and treat impulsivity in personality pathology points to potentially differential mechanisms underlying impulsivity in personality disorder compared to other behavioral expressions of impulsivity and highlights the relationship between impulsivity and suicidal behavior (Linhartová et al., 2020). This relationship can be partially explained because impulsivity profiles in personality disorder appear to be consistently related to situations involving intense negative affect, which is, for example, a different profile when compared to impulsivity in people diagnosed with ADHD (Kenézlői et al., 2022). The role of negative emotion may be one of the pathways connecting different disorders around the expression of impulsive behavior and is likely an adequate model to understand impulsivity and reckless behavior in the setting of personality disorder (Allen et al., 2022).

4.1.2 Aggressive Behavior and the Concept of Dual-Harm

Aggressive behavior has received significant attention in the study of personality pathology, and connections to self-harm and suicidal behavior as a form of aggressive conduct are typically at the center of this clinical and scientific attention. This is particularly true in the case of BPD (Newhill et al., 2009) and ASPD (Jones et al., 2011). However, different pathways have been examined for these two very different expressions of personality pathology. In BPD, trait impulsivity has been consistently related to self-harm and aggressive behavior (Terzi et al., 2017). In a prospective study, Stepp and colleagues (2012) showed that interpersonal problems mediated the relationship between BPD symptoms and violent behaviors, and Candini and colleagues (2020) showed that poor metacognitive functioning (i.e., deficits in an individual's ability to recognize and understand internal states) predicted a history of violent conduct in patients. In ASPD, pathways toward aggression seem to be at least partially related to decreased cognitive (rather than affective) empathy (Waller et al., 2020) and to specific deficits in mentalizing (Falcao et al., 2022). Even though difficulties in empathy and mentalizing are also hallmarks of BPD, in BPD rather than in ASPD, aggressive behavior associated with these deficits is typically reactive rather than proactive (Herpertz et al., 2021). Thus, evidence points to different pathways toward aggressive behavior across different expressions of personality disorder, suggesting nuanced mechanisms and risk factors.

Aggressive behavior has been theoretically and empirically connected to self-harm in personality disorders. BPD traits seem to play a crucial role in the relationships between aggressive behavior and self-harm in a recent network analysis (Nelson et al., 2022). This idea of dual-harm (i.e., harm directed toward the self and others) has been related to a more comprehensive model connecting personality, aggression, and suicidal behaviors. The cognitive-emotional model of dual-harm integrates elements from the General Aggression Model (GAM; Anderson & Bushman, 2002) and diathesis-stress theories, proposing a framework that explains the co-occurrence of self-harm and aggression (Ferguson & Dyck, 2012). It highlights both distal and proximal processes in dual-harm behavior. Distal processes involve biological and environmental factors that shape personality traits, particularly those related to emotional and interpersonal instability. These traits create a predisposition toward harmful behaviors. Proximal processes are more immediate, involving emotional dysregulation and interpersonal motivations as key functions of dual-harm. Individuals may use self-harm and aggression interchangeably as coping mechanisms for distressing emotions or social interactions. Feedback mechanisms reinforce these behaviors by perpetuating maladaptive schemas through negative experiences and environmental responses. This model suggests that interventions should address emotional regulation, maladaptive schemas, and the underlying personality traits to effectively reduce dual-harm behavior (Shafti et al., 2021).

4.1.3 Suicidal Ideation, Suicide Attempts, and NSSI in Personality Disorders: The Dual-System Model

Personality, and precisely personality traits such as neuroticism, hopelessness, and extroversion, have been systematically correlated with suicidal ideation, suicide attempts, and death by suicide (Brezo et al., 2006). In addition to personality traits, emotional dysregulation and negative affect have been consistently used to explain the emergence of behavioral dysregulation and its correlates in suicidal ideation and behavior in personality disorders. However, most studies exploring this association have used cross-sectional designs, so causality cannot be reliably inferred (Turton et al., 2021). In studies that use intensive longitudinal assessment and are thus better suited to explore causality, negative affect as well as interpersonal problems and maladaptive coping (i.e., rumination) have been causally linked to suicidal ideation and self-harm in daily life (Gee et al., 2020). Studies that rely on intensive longitudinal data have also facilitated more nuanced models of ideation-to-action phenomena (i.e., how suicidal ideation is transferred to self-harm, including NSSI, attempts, and death by suicide). The Dual-System Model of Suicidality (DSMS) is an innovative framework designed to explain the mechanisms behind suicidal thoughts and behaviors (STBs) (Brüdern et al., 2022). The model proposes two primary systems of information processing: the reflective system and the impulsive system (Strack & Deutsch, 2004). The reflective system is associated with deliberate, goal-directed behaviors and is driven by self-regulation processes. It is responsible for higher-order mental functions such as planning and problem-solving, operating through a feedback loop to reduce discrepancies between current states and personal goals. This system's involvement means that suicidal behavior can be seen as a maladaptive coping mechanism when individuals are unable to resolve these discrepancies effectively.

On the other hand, the impulsive system operates quickly and effortlessly, often in response to high stress or negative affect. This system is characterized by bottom-up processing and is not dependent on conscious goals or cognitive resources (Hofmann et al., 2008). It is responsible for spontaneous, emotionally driven behaviors and can override the reflective system when self-regulation resources are depleted. This explains why some suicidal behaviors occur impulsively without premeditation, especially under conditions of acute stress or emotional turmoil. The DSMS highlights the importance of both systems in understanding the complexity of suicidal behavior, offering a more comprehensive approach that includes both planned and impulsive suicidal pathways. In a recent experiment that capitalizes on the DSMS, Cho and Shim (2025) identified different decision-making profiles among participants, revealing significant relationships between decision-making deficits, such as high-risk decision-making and slow decision-making speed, and increased rates of suicidal ideation and suicide attempts. Specifically, individuals in the high-risk decision-making class and those with slower decision-making speeds exhibited higher lifetime suicidal excessive theory of mind ideation and suicide attempts, consistent with DSMS's emphasis on how impulsive processes and self-regulation failures can drive suicidal behavior under high-stress conditions.

4.2 Innovation to the Diagnosis of Personality Disorder

4.2.1 Level of Personality Functioning (LPF; Criterion A): Self and Interpersonal Dysfunction

The Level of Personality Functioning, represented by the entry criterion of the AMPD and the new ICD-11 diagnostic system for personality disorders, assesses disturbances in self (identity and self-direction) and interpersonal (empathy and intimacy) functioning. These disturbances represent a general adaptive failure, meaning that individuals with personality disorders struggle significantly with understanding themselves, maintaining consistent self-identity, setting and pursuing realistic goals, understanding and relating to others, and forming and maintaining healthy relationships (Sharp & Wall, 2021). The exact components and definitions of LPF are summarized in Table 4.1.

The LPF was proposed in Section III of the DSM-5 (APA, 2022) to address the well-established limitations of the categorical system, including significant heterogeneity within each personality disorder category, comorbidity between different personality disorder categories, and comorbidity with several other common mental disorders (Clark, 2007; Krueger et al., 2018). Moreover, factor analytic attempts 10 factors to represent the 10 personality disorders described in Section II of the DSM-5 have not been successful (e.g., Sheets & Craighead, 2007), calling into question the structure of personality pathology as represented in Section II of the DSM-5. In response, the AMPD and the ICD-11 models identify a single severity continuum that defines the features shared by all manifestations of personality pathology, that is, maladaptive self- and interpersonal functioning. It states that regardless of specific presentation (e.g., more antisocial or more borderline or more externalizing or more internalizing), all personality disorders struggle with a sense of self and getting on with others.

For enhancing our understanding and treatment of suicidal behaviors, the LPF is considered a significant innovation. This is because most theories, models, and research on suicidal behavior and self-harm in personality disorder draw on themes of self- and interpersonal functioning. Most notable in this regard is the Interpersonal Theory (IPT; Joiner, 2005) of Suicide which stipulates two primary mechanisms that contribute to the development of suicidal ideation: perceived burdensomeness

Table 4.1 Diagnostic criteria for personality disorder based on the alternative model of personality disorder in DSM-5

Component	Description
Criterion A: Level of personality functioning (LPF)	This criterion assesses the severity of impairment in personality functioning. It includes: – Self: Involves identity (sense of self and self-worth) and self-direction (pursuit of meaningful goals) – Interpersonal: Involves empathy (understanding others' experiences and motivations) and intimacy (maintaining close and meaningful relationships)
Criterion B: Pathological personality traits	This criterion includes specific maladaptive personality traits grouped into five broad domains: – Negative affectivity: Frequent and intense experiences of high levels of negative emotions – Detachment: Avoidance of socio-emotional experiences, including withdrawal and anhedonia – Antagonism: Behaviors that put the individual at odds with others, including manipulativeness and deceitfulness – Disinhibition: Orientation toward immediate gratification, leading to impulsivity and irresponsibility – Psychoticism: Exhibiting odd, unusual behaviors and cognitions, including eccentricity and perceptual dysregulation

and thwarted belongingness. Perceived burdensomeness refers to the incorrect mental calculation of self-liability and self-hate, and thwarted belongingness refers to perceived loneliness, social disconnection, and familial conflict (Chu et al., 2017; Van Orden et al., 2010). Both perceived burdensomeness and thwarted belongingness are combined with hopelessness that either of these negative interpersonal cognitions will subside and result in one's desire to die by suicide.

Recently, IPT was extended with mentalization-based theory to more adequately integrate aspects of self-functioning when thinking about the interpersonal determinants of suicidal behaviors specifically relevant to personality disorder (Balzen & Sharp, 2024). Accordingly, it is argued that an integrated sense of self is foundational for important interpersonal functions such as perspective taking, comprehension of others, and the quality and duration of relationships, and underlying an integrated sense of self is the ability to mentalize the self, that is, to make sense of internal states and to allow for the discovery of important aspects of one's subjective experience, leading to a deeper and broader understanding of the self (Fonagy & Target, 1998). These ideas are very consistent with our earlier discussions of the role of negative affect and emotion regulation in suicidal behavior. It is hard to build a solid and integrated sense of self without the capacity to make sense of emotions and thoughts meaningfully. It becomes easy to turn inward against the self without compassion and understanding for the self. Accordingly, research has shown disturbances in self-function associated with suicide, including associations between identity disturbance/incoherence and suicide severity (Sekowski et al., 2022; Sokol & Eisenheim, 2016), more negative self-concept in suicidal adolescents compared to non-suicidal adolescents (Brunstein-Klomek et al., 2005), and increases in levels of personality pathology and subsequent suicidal ideation severity as a function of identity disturbance.

Additionally, poor self-concept integration and identity incoherence have been linked with NSSI in adults (Taylor et al., 2019) and adolescents (Claes et al., 2014), and LPF is associated with several suicide attempts (Kampe et al., 2018). That mentalizing plays a role in supporting integrated self-function is suggested by Hatkevich et al. (2019), who showed in a series of binary logistic regression analyses significant relations between hypermentalizing (excessive theory of mind) and suicidal ideation in the past 4 weeks and suicide attempt in the past year in a large sample of inpatient adolescents. These results fit with a recent meta-analysis showing significant associations between impaired mentalizing and an increased level of suicidality (Nestor & Sutherland, 2022). Impairments in mentalizing associated with suicidality also appear at the level of neurobiology, with fMRI research indicating distinctions between adults who have attempted suicide and those who have never attempted suicide in neural networks involved in the theory of mind processing (Malhi et al., 2022). Taken together, there is emerging evidence that optimal self-function is critical for protection against suicidal behaviors and attempts and that scaffolding mentalizing capacity in individuals can provide the needed reflective capacity to view the self as benign and others as supportive.

4.2.2 Maladaptive Trait Domains and Facets

The AMPD and ICD-11 diagnostic systems allow further specification of the manifestation of personality pathology in individuals by offering clinicians the option to evaluate an individual's level of maladaptive traits. Specific maladaptive traits cut across five broad domains: negative affectivity, detachment, antagonism, disinhibition, and psychoticism. These traits describe the specific ways in which personality disorders manifest but do not alone constitute a personality disorder without the presence of significant impairment in personality functioning, as described in LPF (Clark & Watson, 2022). Suicidal behaviors are explicitly represented in the trait domain of Negative Affectivity, defined thus in the AMPD: "Frequent and intense experiences of high levels of a wide range of negative emotions (e.g., anxiety, depression, guilt/shame, worry, anger) and their behavioral (e.g., self-harm) and interpersonal (e.g., dependency) manifestations." As per the literature reviewed earlier, another relevant trait domain for suicidal behaviors is disinhibition, defined thus in the AMPD: "Orientation toward immediate gratification, leading to impulsive behavior driven by current thoughts, feelings, and external stimuli, without regard for past learning or consideration of future consequences." Further, the trait facet of depressiveness includes an explicit reference to suicidal behaviors: "Feelings of being down, miserable, and/or hopeless; difficulty recovering from such moods; pessimism about the future; pervasive shame and/or guilt; feelings of inferior self-worth; thoughts of suicide and suicidal behavior." Given this explicit inclusion of suicidal behaviors, it is not surprising that maladaptive trait domains are associated with self-harm (e.g., Somma et al., 2019). Especially the detachment domain appears to predict lethality in suicide attempts (Borroni et al., 2023), suggesting an intensely interpersonal function of actual suicide attempts.

4.3 Suicidal Behavior as a Correlate to Severity across Mental Disorders

All mental health disorders are associated with a higher risk of suicidal behavior, and most suicide attempts and deaths by suicides occur in persons with a mental health disorder (Too et al., 2019). This stable finding suggests that suicidal behavior is a transdiagnostic phenomenon with shared mechanisms. Evidence regarding the transdiagnostic nature of mechanisms underpinning suicidal behaviors is relevant, and current hierarchical models of psychopathology are better suited to accommodate transdiagnostic features, including suicidal behavior (Lahey et al., 2021).

4.3.1 Evidence Suggesting Shared Transdiagnostic Mechanisms of Suicidal Behavior

Suicide remains a significant public health crisis, with recent efforts focused on understanding the complex interplay of factors contributing to suicidal behavior. Recent research on suicidal behavior highlights the importance of understanding it as a transdiagnostic phenomenon intersecting with various mental health disorders and conditions. Several mechanisms related to suicidal behaviors, including ideation, attempts, NSSI, and death by suicide, have been examined in recent years, providing promising directions in the study of the transdiagnostic nature of suicidal behaviors.

The stress-diathesis model is central to this understanding, positing that while psychiatric disorders significantly contribute to suicide risk, they do not fully account for suicidality. This model incorporates a diathesis—vulnerability, including factors such as impulsivity and aggressive traits—that interacts with stressors to elevate suicide risk. Several identified mechanisms can be understood from the perspective of individual vulnerabilities (Sisti et al., 2020).

Chronic pain provides a salient example of the transdiagnostic nature of suicidal behavior. Individuals with chronic pain experience significantly higher rates of suicidal ideation and behavior compared to the general population. This elevated risk is not merely due to the presence of pain but is intricately linked to several psychological processes. Perceived burdensomeness, as mentioned earlier, and thwarted belongingness, an unmet need for social connection, are significant factors contributing to suicidality in chronic pain patients (Kirtley et al., 2020). When chronic pain correlates with mental defeat, negative beliefs about the self, and chronic or persistent stressors, the risk is further compounded. Indeed, mental defeat is strongly associated with the worst-ever suicidal intent, surpassing the impact of other factors such as anxiety and depression (Kirtley et al., 2020).

Psychological flexibility is another transdiagnostic factor relevant to suicidality, particularly in individuals exposed to early-life maltreatment (Türk et al., 2024). Psychological flexibility involves staying present with distressing experiences and pursuing valued life goals despite these challenges. Higher levels of psychological flexibility are associated with lower levels of depression and pain over time, indicating its protective role against suicidal ideation. This concept underscores the importance of fostering psychological resilience and adaptability to mitigate suicide risk across various mental health conditions (Kirtley et al., 2020).

Future orientation and self-regulation are also pivotal in the transdiagnostic understanding of suicidal behavior. Difficulties in maintaining positive future thinking and self-regulation are common in individuals with personality disorders and significantly contribute to suicidal ideation. The struggle to reconcile current self-perceptions with ideal self-representations can exacerbate psychological distress and increase suicide risk. Addressing these cognitive patterns through targeted interventions can help reduce suicidality in individuals dealing with chronic pain and other psychiatric disorders (Lind et al., 2020).

Several other underpinnings of suicidal behavior have been identified that are shared across mental disorders, including interpersonal factors such as perceived burdensomeness and thwarted belongingness (Jacobucci et al., 2023), along with cognitive factors such as hopelessness, mental pain, and intolerance to suffering (Landi et al., 2021). Impaired cognitive control, especially in decision-making, further exacerbates the risk of severe suicide attempts (Sastre-Buades et al., 2021), and the interaction of genetic vulnerability and environmental stressors, as explained by stress-diathesis dynamics, plays a crucial role in the development of suicidal behaviors (Steinberg & Mann, 2020). Regarding environmental stressors, recent research has pointed to the mediating role of impulsivity in the relationship between childhood maltreatment and suicidal behavior (Pérez-Balaguer et al., 2022).

In conclusion, the transdiagnostic perspective on suicidal behavior underscores the complex interplay of various psychological factors across different mental health conditions. By recognizing suicidal behavior as a distinct psychopathological domain and addressing transdiagnostic factors such as perceived burdensomeness, mental defeat, psychological flexibility, and future orientation, researchers and clinicians can develop more effective interventions and prevention strategies. This holistic approach is essential for reducing the global burden of suicide and improving outcomes for individuals at risk.

4.3.2 Suicidal Behavior in the Context of Hierarchical Models of Psychopathology

Hierarchical models of psychopathology have emerged as a transformative framework for understanding mental disorders (Lahey et al., 2021). These models conceptualize psychopathology as consisting of continuous dimensions rather than discrete categories, challenging traditional diagnostic systems like the DSM and ICD. The Hierarchical Taxonomy of Psychopathology (HiTOP) is a prominent example, proposing a multitiered structure where broad higher-order factors, such as internalizing and externalizing dimensions, encompass narrower syndromes and specific symptoms (Ringwald et al., 2023). The hierarchical approach offers significant advantages in capturing the complexity of mental health disorders (Markon, 2021). It recognizes that different mental disorders often share features, leading to high comorbidity rates. For instance, anxiety and depression frequently co-occur and share underlying risk factors, which a higher-order internalizing factor in the HiTOP model can represent. This model posits a general factor of psychopathology, often called the "p factor," which captures the common variance across various mental disorders (Caspi et al., 2014; Fried et al., 2021). Studies have shown that this general factor is highly predictive of functional outcomes such as psychiatric hospitalization, treatment needs, and overall disability, even though recently, the concept has received criticism for equating statistical model fit with validity (Watts et al., 2024).

Understanding suicidal behavior through the lens of hierarchical models highlights its transdiagnostic nature. Suicidal behavior often coexists with various mental health conditions, including mood disorders, anxiety disorders, substance use disorders, and personality disorders (Krueger et al., 2021). By focusing on underlying dimensions rather than specific diagnostic categories, hierarchical models can better identify individuals at risk of suicide. The "p factor" in these models encompasses a range of emotional and behavioral dysregulations that are commonly associated with increased suicide risk. For example, individuals with high scores on the general factor of psychopathology are more likely to experience severe and persistent distress, impulsivity, and poor emotion regulation, all of which are critical risk factors for suicidal behavior (Lahey et al., 2021). Hierarchical models are particularly relevant for understanding and treating personality disorders due to their dimensional nature but provide a general framework to understand co-occurrence and co-variance across mental disorders (Widiger, Bach, et al., 2019). Traditional diagnostic systems often struggle with the overlap and comorbidity among personality disorders (Widiger, Sellbom, et al., 2019). HiTOP and similar models provide a more nuanced understanding by situating personality pathology within a broader spectrum of psychopathology. This approach allows for identifying shared and unique features across different personality disorders. For instance, traits such as emotional instability and impulsivity, common in BPD, can be understood as part of broader internalizing and externalizing dimensions. This perspective facilitates targeted interventions that address the specific symptoms of personality disorders and the broader underlying dimensions (Kotov et al., 2017). Integrating hierarchical models into clinical practice holds promise for improving the diagnosis and treatment of mental disorders. By moving away from rigid categorical diagnoses, clinicians can adopt a more flexible, individualized approach that considers the full spectrum of a patient's psychopathology (Ringwald et al., 2023). This can lead to more effective treatment plans that address the specific and general aspects of a patient's mental health. Moreover, these models can guide the development of new therapeutic interventions that target the underlying dimensions of psychopathology, potentially leading to more robust and lasting improvements in mental health outcomes (Ruggero et al., 2019).

Hierarchical models of psychopathology represent a significant advance in our understanding of mental disorders and their interrelationships. By emphasizing the dimensional and transdiagnostic nature of psychopathology, these models offer a more comprehensive framework for understanding and treating mental health issues, including suicidal behavior. Their relevance to personality disorders underscores the potential for hierarchical models to transform clinical practice and improve patient care.

4.3.3 Suicidal Behaviors and Personality Disorders in the Context of the RDoC Framework

Cognitive system domains provide essential insights into understanding suicidal behaviors, mainly through the constructs of attention, cognitive control, declarative and working memory, language, and perception (Huber et al., 2019). Studies reviewed under the Research Domain Criteria (RDoC) framework have shown significant differences in cognitive control between individuals with suicidal behaviors and both patient and healthy controls. Cognitive control deficits, including impaired response inhibition and cognitive flexibility, are notably prevalent in those with suicidal ideation and attempts. These impairments may contribute to the progression from ideation to attempts, especially more lethal or violent attempts (Glenn et al., 2017). Additionally, deficits in declarative and working memory are associated with the severity of suicidal attempts, indicating that cognitive dysfunction plays a crucial role in suicidal behavior. These cognitive deficits often coexist with various psychiatric disorders, such as depression, bipolar disorder, and schizophrenia, suggesting that addressing cognitive impairments could be integral to understanding and preventing suicidal behaviors among individuals with personality disorders (Bredemeier & Miller, 2015).

Negative Valence System domains have also been related to increased risk for suicidal behaviors, especially in the context of personality disorders. Negative Valence Systems encompass responses to aversive situations and stimuli, including fear, anxiety, and loss, which are closely linked to emotional dysregulation seen in personality disorders (Koudys et al., 2019). For instance, hopelessness and rumination, both key Negative Valence System constructs, are strongly associated with suicidal ideation and attempts. Individuals with personality disorders, particularly BPD, exhibit heightened sensitivity to these negative valence stimuli, leading to intense emotional reactions and impulsivity that elevate suicide risk (Koudys et al., 2019). Dysfunction in Negative Valence Systems can result in persistent negative emotional states, reinforcing maladaptive coping mechanisms like self-harm and suicidal behavior. Understanding these Negative Valence System mechanisms provides a nuanced perspective on the interplay between emotional regulation deficits and suicide risk in personality disorders (Glenn et al., 2018).

The regulatory and arousal systems, along with social processes domains, are intricately linked to suicidal behaviors and NSSI in individuals with personality disorders (Schreiner et al., 2015). The arousal system, which encompasses circadian rhythms and sleep-wakefulness, influences emotional reactivity and regulation (Fernandez et al., 2016). Dysregulation in these systems can lead to heightened sensitivity to stressors and impaired coping mechanisms, contributing to the propensity for NSSI and suicidal behaviors (Schreiner et al., 2015). For instance, disturbances in sleep patterns and circadian rhythms have been associated with an increased risk of depression and NSSI, highlighting the critical role of regulatory systems in emotional stability (Arns et al., 2015). Additionally, the social processes domain, which includes constructs like affiliation and attachment, social communication, and perception and understanding of self and others, plays a significant role in these behaviors (Clarkson et al., 2020). Individuals with personality disorders often experience difficulties in these areas, such as heightened rejection sensitivity and impaired self-other conceptualizations, which can exacerbate stress and emotional dysregulation, leading to NSSI and suicidal tendencies (Hanegraaf et al., 2021; Stewart et al., 2019). These findings underscore the importance of addressing both arousal/regulatory and social processes in understanding and treating suicidal behaviors in this population.

4.4 Suicidal Behavior in Personality Disorders from the Lens of Current Theoretical Models for Suicidality

There are currently several models to explain suicidal behavior from a transdiagnostic approach. Some of these models provide important mechanisms that help clarify suicidal behavior in persons diagnosed with personality disorders. We summarize current models that have grown out of scientific evidence and reflect on their implications for understanding suicidality in personality disorders.

4.4.1 Integrated Motivational-Volitional Model

This model has been proposed by O'Connor and Kirtley (2018). The integrated motivational-volitional (IMV) model of suicidal behavior offers a comprehensive framework to understand the progression from suicidal ideation to suicidal actions, emphasizing the roles of defeat, entrapment, and volitional moderators. Although this is a transdiagnostic model, the IMV model is particularly relevant in the context of personality disorders as conceptualized by the AMPD, which highlights impairments in self- and interpersonal functioning. The IMV model's emphasis on psychological processes like defeat and entrapment aligns closely with the AMPD's focus on the chronic, pervasive negative emotional states and impaired coping mechanisms seen in personality disorders, mainly as related to interpersonal stress and self-concept dysregulation (Souza et al., 2024). Individuals with personality disorders often experience heightened vulnerability to feelings of defeat and entrapment, which can exacerbate suicidal ideation, according to the IMV. Loneliness, experiential avoidance, and rigid perfectionism conceptualized in the ICD-11 as anankastic have been studied in relationship with de IMV and are also prevalent in individuals experiencing personality disorders (McClelland et al., 2021; Ordóñez-Carrasco et al., 2020). Moreover, the volitional phase of the IMV model, which includes factors such as impulsivity, access to means, and exposure to suicidal behavior, is critical in understanding why some individuals with personality disorders progress from ideation to suicidal action, particularly those with a phenotype characterized by increase impulsivity (Kaurin et al., 2022). The AMPD framework, with its focus on core impairments and maladaptive traits, provides a rich context for applying the IMV model, particularly in identifying those at the highest risk for transitioning from suicidal thoughts to attempts with many of its components closely aligning with evidence on suicidal behavior in personality disorder (McClelland et al., 2023). This integration underscores the importance of targeted interventions that address both the motivational and volitional factors in this population, potentially reducing the incidence of suicide among those with severe personality pathology.

4.4.2 Interpersonal Theory

The interpersonal theory of suicide, as proposed by Joiner and colleagues (2009), suggests that suicidal behavior arises when individuals simultaneously experience two critical psychological states: perceived burdensomeness (the belief that one is a burden to others) and thwarted belongingness (a profound sense of alienation and lack of connection with others). These states create a desire for death, but for a person to act on this desire, they must also possess the capability for suicide, which is acquired over time through habituation to painful or fear-inducing experiences, such as previous self-harm or exposure to violence.

In the context of personality disorders, particularly those conceptualized through the AMPD, this theory offers significant insights. Individuals with personality disorders often exhibit chronic patterns of interpersonal dysfunction, including difficulties in forming and maintaining relationships, which can exacerbate feelings of thwarted belongingness (Dienst et al., 2023). Additionally, traits such as emotional dysregulation, impulsivity, and a history of trauma or self-harm, common in many personality disorders, can contribute to both perceived burdensomeness and the acquired capability for suicide. The implication is that therapeutic interventions for individuals with personality disorders should focus on addressing these interpersonal deficits and the distorted self-perceptions that contribute to suicidal ideation (Rogers & Joiner Jr, 2016). Enhancing social connectedness, challenging perceptions of burdensomeness, and reducing exposure to situations that could further habituate the individual to self-harm are critical strategies. By integrating the interpersonal theory with the AMPD framework, clinicians can better understand and mitigate the risk factors for suicidality in this vulnerable population.

4.4.3 Three-Step Theory

The three-step theory of suicide, developed by Klonsky and May (2015), presents a streamlined model within the "ideation-to-action" framework that explains the development of suicidal ideation and the progression to suicide attempts. The theory consists of three key steps:

1. Development of suicidal ideation: The first step posits that suicidal ideation arises when an individual experiences a combination of psychological pain (which can be emotional or physical) and hopelessness. This combination is crucial, as pain alone does not typically lead to suicidal thoughts unless accompanied by a sense of hopelessness that the pain will never improve.
2. Escalation of suicidal ideation: The second step involves the role of connectedness as a protective factor. Connectedness refers to an individual's attachment to others, roles, or life purposes. When connectedness is greater than the individual's pain, suicidal ideation remains moderate. However, if connectedness is weaker than the pain and hopelessness, suicidal ideation can intensify.

3. Progression from ideation to attempt: The final step examines why some individuals with strong suicidal ideation go on to make suicide attempts. This progression is influenced by three types of contributors to suicide capacity: dispositional factors (such as genetic predispositions to low pain sensitivity), acquired factors (such as habituation to pain or fear through experiences like self-harm), and practical factors (such as access to means of suicide). An individual with intense suicidal ideation is more likely to attempt suicide if they possess these capabilities.

In the context of personality disorders, which are characterized by chronic emotional instability, interpersonal difficulties, and often a history of trauma or self-harm, the three-step theory has significant implications. Individuals with personality disorders are more likely to experience the psychological pain and hopelessness described in the first step of the three-step theory (Salsman & Linehan, 2012). Furthermore, their often tenuous social connections may diminish the protective factor of connectedness, leading to a heightened risk of severe suicidal ideation (Tsai et al., 2021). The history of impulsivity, self-harm, or exposure to trauma common in personality disorders also contributes to the acquired capability for suicide, making the transition from ideation to action more likely (Kaurin et al., 2022). Therefore, the three-step theory suggests that interventions for suicidality in individuals with personality disorders should focus on reducing psychological pain, fostering hope, strengthening social connectedness and decreasing interpersonal hypersensitivity, and addressing the practical and acquired capacities for suicide.

4.4.4 Suicide Crisis Syndrome

The suicide crisis syndrome (SCS) is a concept developed by Galynker and colleagues (2017) that captures an acute psychological state believed to precede suicidal behavior immediately. It is characterized by intense feelings and cognitive disruptions, including a profound sense of entrapment, where individuals feel completely trapped in their situation with no perceived way out. This is often accompanied by panic and dissociative experiences, where a person might feel disconnected from reality or experience intense fear, sometimes to the point of panic attacks (Schuck et al., 2019). Alongside these symptoms is ruminative flooding, where the individual is overwhelmed by uncontrollable, repetitive thoughts that exacerbate feelings of despair and hopelessness. The emotional pain associated with this state is described as excruciating and unbearable, pushing the person toward considering suicide as a means of escape.

Additionally, there is often an acute fear of dying, which paradoxically intensifies the emotional turmoil but also reflects the severity of the crisis. In the context of personality disorders, especially those characterized by chronic emotional dysregulation and impulsivity, the implications of the SCS are particularly significant. Individuals with personality disorders frequently experience intense emotional pain and feelings of entrapment, making them more susceptible to entering this acute suicidal state (Salsman & Linehan, 2012). For example, in BPD, the combination of extreme emotional sensitivity, interpersonal rejection, and chronic feelings of emptiness can align closely with the components of the SCS, particularly during moments of acute stress or interpersonal conflict (Yen et al., 2021). This makes the SCS a valuable framework for understanding and predicting suicidal behavior in this population, as traditional risk factors may not capture the immediate risk posed by these acute psychological states (Flint et al., 2021).

4.5 Current Findings Regarding Cultural Variability in Suicidal Behavior in Personality Disorder

A good understanding of cultural variability in suicidal behavior in personality disorder is impeded by the variation in the quality of data on suicidal behaviors as well as the general paucity of research in some of the most populous countries of the world in Asia and other regions. Data is even scarcer for suicidal behaviors in the context of personality disorder specifically. In both cases, most of what we know about suicide and personality disorder comes from Western, Educated, Industrial, Rich and Democratic (WEIRD) countries. Social structural adversity, such as exposure to violence, childhood abuse, and privation, as well as intractable social problems, have all been shown to increase the risk of suicidal behavior (Kirmayer, 2022). However, these structural and systemic issues are underwritten by cultural values, institutions, and practices and are thus mediated by cultural meanings and contexts (Kirmayer, 2022). For instance, in a recent study utilizing cultural consensus modeling to understand better the reasons for suicidal behaviors among Black youth, Hill et al. (2025) showed that racism trumped other well-known reasons for suicide among Black youth. In a thoughtful review of how culture may mediate suicidal behaviors, Kirmayer (2022) listed the main identified mechanisms for suicidal behaviors across different theories and models, some of which we also highlighted in this chapter and suggested specific cultural mediators for consideration. These are summarized in Table 4.2.

We are unaware of any research that attempts to integrate some of the social factors and cultural mediators in a personality disorder context and view such integrative research as a critical avenue for future research.

4.6 Implications for Research and Clinical Practice

This chapter has examined the intricate relationship between suicidal behavior and personality disorders, emphasizing the significant role of behavioral dysregulation, impulsivity, emotional dysregulation, and interpersonal functioning in the manifestation of suicidal ideation and attempts. The transdiagnostic nature of these behaviors suggests that while certain features, such as impulsivity and aggressive

Table 4.2 Psychosocial factors and cultural components and mechanisms of suicidal behavior

Psychosocial factor	Cultural component
Intense pain and dysphoria	Societal attitudes toward pain, suffering, and coping strategies
Experience of failure, defeat, shame, and humiliation	Cultural expectations for achievement, perceptions of failure, and codes of honor
Lack of connectedness, social withdrawal, isolation, loneliness	Social norms around age and gender roles, types of relationships, and social networks
Sense of not belonging, social exclusion	Cultural constructions of identity and social participation practices
Perception of being a burden on others	Cultural expectations regarding age, gender, autonomy and contributions to family and community
Racism and discrimination	Cultural interpretations of racial identities
Excessive regulation, rigid social structures	Cultural views on social hierarchy and expectations for conformity
Entrapment	Societal mobility, flexibility in negotiating roles, and opportunities for challenging intolerable situations
Idea of suicide	Cultural models, beliefs, and meanings attributed to suicide
Exposure to media representations of suicide	Cultural constructions of identity, media consumption habits, and prevalence of role models
Availability of means	Cultural attitudes and practices related to firearms, pesticides, medications, and risk-taking behaviors
Capability for suicide	Social modeling of suicidal acts, identification practices, and involvement in risk-taking behaviors

Note: Adapted from Kirmayer (2022)

behavior, are shared across various mental health conditions, they manifest uniquely within the context of personality disorders, particularly in BPD. This uniqueness underscores the importance of tailoring interventions to address the specific mechanisms driving suicidality in these populations, also considering cultural mediators.

The integration of current models of suicidal behavior and specifically of ideation to action pathways needs to be further incorporated into the AMPD to produce a nuanced understanding of how suicidal behaviors develop and persist in individuals with personality dysfunction. The emphasis on impaired self- and interpersonal functioning within the AMPD aligns with the psychological processes identified in these models, such as defeat, entrapment, and emotional dysregulation, which are particularly pronounced in personality disorders.

Future research should continue to explore the intersection of personality pathology and suicidal behavior, mainly through longitudinal studies that can better capture the dynamic nature of these risks. Additionally, given the cultural variability in the expression and recognition of personality disorders and suicidal behavior, it is imperative to develop culturally sensitive diagnostic and intervention strategies that can more effectively address the global burden of these conditions. By focusing on both the transdiagnostic and disorder-specific aspects of suicidality, clinicians can develop more comprehensive and effective prevention and treatment approaches, ultimately reducing the incidence of suicide among individuals with personality disorders.

References

Allen, T. A., Hallquist, M. N., Wright, A. G., & Dombrovski, A. Y. (2022). Negative affectivity and disinhibition as moderators of an interpersonal pathway to suicidal behavior in borderline personality disorder. *Clinical Psychological Science, 10*(5), 856–868. https://doi.org/10.1177/21677026211056686

American Psychiatric Association (APA). (2022). Diagnostic and statistical manual of mental disorders (5th ed., text rev.; DSM-5-TR). American Psychiatric Publishing.

Anderson, C. A., & Bushman, B. J. (2002). Human aggression. *Annual Review of Psychology, 53*(1), 27–51. https://doi.org/10.1146/annurev.psych.53.100901.135231

Arns, M., Swatzyna, R. J., Gunkelman, J., & Olbrich, S. (2015). Sleep maintenance, spindling excessive beta and impulse control: An RDoC arousal and regulatory systems approach? *Neuropsychiatric Electrophysiology, 1*, 1–11. https://doi.org/10.1186/s40810-015-0005-9

Arsenault-Lapierre, G., Kim, C., & Turecki, G. (2004). Psychiatric diagnoses in 3275 suicides: a meta-analysis. *BMC psychiatry, 4*, 1–11. https://doi.org/10.1186/1471-244X-4-37

Balzen, K. M., & Sharp, C. (2024). The contribution of mentalization-based theory and practice for understanding and treating self-injurious behavior in young people. *Journal of Infant, Child, and Adolescent Psychotherapy, 23*(1), 108–121. https://doi-org.pucdechile.idm.oclc.org/10.1080/15289168.2024.2311555

Benton, T. D., Muhrer, E., Jones, J. D., & Lewis, J. (2021). Dysregulation and suicide in children and adolescents. *Child and Adolescent Psychiatric Clinics, 30*(2), 389–399. https://doi.org/10.1016/j.chc.2020.10.008

Borroni, S., Franchini, L., Brioschi, S., Vassena, G., Masci, E., Franzoni, C., et al. (2023). The role of clinical and personological features in predicting high lethality suicide attempts: A study among mood disorder patients. *Personality and Mental Health, 17*(1), 99–106. https://doi.org/10.1002/pmh.1546

Bredemeier, K., & Miller, I. W. (2015). Executive function and suicidality: A systematic qualitative review. *Clinical Psychology Review, 40*, 170–183. https://doi-org.pucdechile.idm.oclc.org/10.1016/j.cpr.2015.06.005

Brezo, J., Paris, J., & Turecki, G. (2006). Personality traits as correlates of suicidal ideation, suicide attempts, and suicide completions: A systematic review. *Acta Psychiatrica Scandinavica, 113*(3), 180–206. https://doi.org/10.1111/j.1600-0447.2005.00702.x

Brüdern, J., Glaesmer, H., Berger, T., & Spangenberg, L. (2022). Understanding suicidal pathways through the lens of a Dual-System Model of Suicidality in real-time: The potential of ecological momentary assessments. *Frontiers in Psychiatry, 13*, 899500. https://doi.org/10.3389/fpsyt.2022.899500

Brunstein-Klomek, A., Orbach, I., Meged, S., & Zalsman, G. (2005). Self complexity of suicidal adolescents. *International Journal of Adolescent Medicine and Health, 17*(3), 267–273.

Candini, V., Ghisi, M., Bianconi, G., Bulgari, V., Carcione, A., Cavalera, C., ... & VIORMED-2 Group Stefano Barlati Assunta Martinazzoli Giuliana Mina Roberta Paleari Francesco Restaino Bruno Travasso Antonio Vita. (2020). Aggressive behavior and metacognitive functions: a longitudinal study on patients with mental disorders. *Annals of general psychiatry, 19*, 1–13. https://doi.org/10.1186/s12991-020-00286-3.

Caspi, A., Houts, R. M., Belsky, D. W., Goldman-Mellor, S. J., Harrington, H., Israel, S., et al. (2014). The p factor: One general psychopathology factor in the structure of psychiatric disorders? *Clinical Psychological Science, 2*(2), 119–137. https://doi.org/10.1177/2167702613497473

Cho, D., & Shim, E. J. (2025). Profiles of decision-making and suicidal behaviors. *Archives of suicide research, 29*(1), 103–117. https://doi.org/10.1080/13811118.2024.2324974

Chu, C., Buchman-Schmitt, J. M., Stanley, I. H., Hom, M. A., Tucker, R. P., Hagan, C. R., ... & Joiner Jr, T. E. (2017). The interpersonal theory of suicide: A systematic review and meta-analysis of a decade of cross-national research. *Psychological bulletin, 143*(12), 1313. https://doi.org/10.1037/bul0000123

Claes, L., Luyckx, K., & Bijttebier, P. (2014). Non-suicidal self-injury in adolescents: Prevalence and associations with identity formation above and beyond depression. *Personality and Individual Differences, 61*, 101–104. https://doi.org/10.1016/j.paid.2013.12.019

Clark, L. A. (2007). Assessment and diagnosis of personality disorder: Perennial issues and an emerging reconceptualization. *Annual Review of Psychology, 58*, 227–257. https://doi.org/10.1146/annurev.psych.57.102904.190200

Clark, L. A., & Watson, D. (2022). The trait model of the DSM–5 alternative model of personality disorder (AMPD): A structural review. *Personality Disorders: Theory, Research, and Treatment, 13*(4), 328–336. https://doi.org/10.1037/per0000568.supp

Clarkson, T., Kang, E., Capriola-Hall, N., Lerner, M. D., Jarcho, J., & Prinstein, M. J. (2020). Meta-analysis of the RDoC social processing domain across units of analysis in children and adolescents. *Journal of Clinical Child & Adolescent Psychology, 49*(3), 297–321. https://doi.org/10.1080/15374416.2019.1678167

de la Torre-Luque, A., Pemau, A., Ayad-Ahmed, W., Borges, G., Fernandez-Sevillano, J., Garrido-Torres, N., ... & Survive Consortium. (2023). Risk of suicide attempt repetition after an index attempt: A systematic review and meta-analysis. General hospital psychiatry, 81, 51–56. https://doi.org/10.1016/j.genhosppsych.2023.01.007

Dienst, F., Forkmann, T., Schreiber, D., & Höller, I. (2023). Attachment and need to belong as moderators of the relationship between thwarted belongingness and suicidal ideation. *BMC Psychology, 11*(1), 50. https://doi.org/10.1186/s40359-023-01080-y

Ditrich, I., Philipsen, A., & Matthies, S. (2021). Borderline personality disorder (BPD) and attention deficit hyperactivity disorder (ADHD) revisited–a review-update on common grounds and subtle distinctions. *Borderline Personality Disorder and Emotion Dysregulation, 8*, 1–12. https://doi.org/10.1186/s40479-021-00162-w

Falcao, V., Pinto, C., & Heitor, M. J. (2022). Antisocial personality disorder: What else can be done? *European Psychiatry, 65*(S1), S667–S668. https://doi.org/10.1192/j.eurpsy.2022.1716

Ferguson, C. J., & Dyck, D. (2012). Paradigm change in aggression research: The time has come to retire the General Aggression Model. *Aggression and Violent Behavior, 17*(3), 220–228. https://doi.org/10.1016/j.avb.2012.02.007

Fernandez, K. C., Jazaieri, H., & Gross, J. J. (2016). Emotion regulation: A transdiagnostic perspective on a new RDoC domain. *Cognitive Therapy and Research, 40*, 426–440. https://doi.org/10.1007/s10608-016-9772-2

Flint, J., Cohen, L., Nath, D., Habib, Z., Guo, X., Galynker, I., & Calati, R. (2021). The association between the suicide crisis syndrome and suicidal behaviors: The moderating role of personality traits. *European Psychiatry, 64*(1), e63. https://doi.org/10.1192/j.eurpsy.2021.2235

Fried, E. I., Greene, A. L., & Eaton, N. R. (2021). The p factor is the sum of its parts, for now. *World Psychiatry, 20*(1), 69. https://doi.org/10.1002/wps.20814

Fonagy, P., & Target, M. (1998). Mentalization and the changing aims of child psychoanalysis. *Psychoanalytic dialogues, 8*(1), 87–114. https://doi.org/10.1080/10481889809539235

Galynker, I., Yaseen, Z. S., Cohen, A., Benhamou, O., Hawes, M., & Briggs, J. (2017). Prediction of suicidal behavior in high risk psychiatric patients using an assessment of acute suicidal state: the suicide crisis inventory. *Depression and anxiety, 34*(2), 147–158. https://doi.org/10.1002/da.22559

Gee, B. L., Han, J., Benassi, H., & Batterham, P. J. (2020). Suicidal thoughts, suicidal behaviours and self-harm in daily life: A systematic review of ecological momentary assessment studies. *Digital Health, 6*, 2055207620963958. https://doi.org/10.1177/2055207620963958

Glenn, J. J., Werntz, A. J., Slama, S. J., Steinman, S. A., Teachman, B. A., & Nock, M. K. (2017). Suicide and self-injury-related implicit cognition: A large-scale examination and replication. *Journal of abnormal psychology, 126*(2), 199. https://doi.org/10.1037/abn0000230

Glenn, C. R., Kleiman, E. M., Cha, C. B., Deming, C. A., Franklin, J. C., & Nock, M. K. (2018). Understanding suicide risk within the Research Domain Criteria (RDoC) framework: A meta-analytic review. *Depression and Anxiety, 35*(1), 65–88. https://doi.org/10.1002/da.22686

Hanegraaf, L., van Baal, S., Hohwy, J., & Verdejo-Garcia, A. (2021). A systematic review and meta-analysis of 'Systems for Social Processes' in borderline personality and substance use disorders. *Neuroscience & Biobehavioral Reviews, 127*, 572–592. https://doi.org/10.1016/j.neubiorev.2021.04.013

Hatkevich, C., Venta, A., & Sharp, C. (2019). Theory of mind and suicide ideation and attempt in adolescent inpatients. *Journal of Affective Disorders, 256*, 17–25. https://doi.org/10.1016/j.jad.2019.05.051

Herpertz, S. C., Matzke, B., Hillmann, K., Neukel, C., Mancke, F., Jaentsch, B., et al. (2021). A mechanism-based group-psychotherapy approach to aggressive behaviour in borderline personality disorder: Findings from a cluster-randomised controlled trial. *BJPsych Open, 7*(1), e17. https://doi.org/10.1192/bjo.2020.131

Hill, R. M., Busby, D., Brown, J. L., Sumlin, E., Fernandez, E., & Sharp, C. (2025). Cultural Consensus Modeling to identify culturally relevant reasons for and against suicide among Black adolescents. *Suicide and Life-Threatening Behavior, 55*(1), e13000. https://doi.org/10.1111/sltb.13000

Hofmann, W., Friese, M., & Wiers, R. W. (2008). Impulsive versus reflective influences on health behavior: A theoretical framework and empirical review. *Health Psychology Review, 2*(2), 111–137. https://doi.org/10.1080/17437190802617668

Huber, R. S., Hodgson, R., & Yurgelun-Todd, D. A. (2019). A qualitative systematic review of suicide behavior using the cognitive systems domain of the research domain criteria (RDoC) framework. *Psychiatry Research, 282*, 112589. https://doi.org/10.1016/j.psychres.2019.112589

Jacobucci, R., McClure, K., & Ammerman, B. A. (2023). Comparing the role of perceived burdensomeness and thwarted belongingness in prospectively predicting active suicidal ideation. *Suicide and Life-threatening Behavior, 53*(2), 198–206. https://doi.org/10.1111/sltb.12933

Joiner, T. (2005). *Why people die by suicide* (Vol. 276). Harvard University Press.

Joiner Jr, T. E., Van Orden, K. A., Witte, T. K., Selby, E. A., Ribeiro, J. D., Lewis, R., & Rudd, M. D. (2009). Main predictions of the interpersonal–psychological theory of suicidal behavior: Empirical tests in two samples of young adults. *Journal of abnormal psychology, 118*(3), 634. https://doi.org/10.1037/a0016500.

Jones, S. E., Miller, J. D., & Lynam, D. R. (2011). Personality, antisocial behavior, and aggression: A meta-analytic review. *Journal of Criminal Justice, 39*(4), 329–337. https://doi.org/10.1016/j.jcrimjus.2011.03.004

Kampe, L., Zimmermann, J., Bender, D., Caligor, E., Borowski, A. L., Ehrenthal, J. C., et al. (2018). Comparison of the structured DSM–5 clinical interview for the level of personality functioning scale with the structured interview of personality organization. *Journal of Personality Assessment, 100*(6), 642–649. https://doi.org/10.1080/00223891.2018.1489257

Kaurin, A., Dombrovski, A. Y., Hallquist, M. N., & Wright, A. G. (2022). Momentary interpersonal processes of suicidal surges in borderline personality disorder. *Psychological Medicine, 52*(13), 2702–2712. https://doi.org/10.1017/S0033291720004791

Kenézlői, E., Balogh, L., Somogyi, S., Lévay, E., Bajzát, B., Halmai, Z., et al. (2022). Comparative analysis of impulsivity profiles in adult attention deficit hyperactivity disorder and borderline personality disorder. *European Psychiatry, 65*(S1), S867–S868. https://doi.org/10.1192/j.eurpsy.2022.2249

Kirmayer, L. J. (2022). Suicide in cultural context: An ecosocial approach. *Transcultural Psychiatry, 59*(1), 3–12. https://doi.org/10.1177/13634615221076424

Kirtley, O. J., Rodham, K., & Crane, C. (2020). Understanding suicidal ideation and behaviour in individuals with chronic pain: A review of the role of novel transdiagnostic psychological factors. *The Lancet Psychiatry, 7*(3), 282–290. https://doi.org/10.1016/S2215-0366(19)30288-3

Klonsky, E. D., & May, A. M. (2015). The three-step theory (3ST): A new theory of suicide rooted in the "ideation-to-action" framework. *International Journal of Cognitive Therapy, 8*(2), 114–129. https://doi.org/10.1521/ijct.2015.8.2.114

Kotov, R., Krueger, R. F., Watson, D., Achenbach, T. M., Althoff, R. R., Bagby, R. M., Brown, T. A., Carpenter, W. T., Caspi, A., Clark, L. A., Eaton, N. R., Forbes, M. K., Forbush, K. T., Goldberg, D., Hasin, D., Hyman, S. E., Ivanova, M. Y., Lynam, D. R., Markon, K., Miller, J. D., et al. (2017). The Hierarchical Taxonomy of Psychopathology (HiTOP): A dimensional alternative to traditional nosologies. *Journal of Abnormal Psychology, 126*(4), 454–477. https://doi.org/10.1037/abn0000258

Koudys, J. W., Cane, C., Nikolova, Y. S., & Ruocco, A. C. (2023). Transdiagnostic impulsivity-relevant phenotypes and the comorbidity of personality disorders with substance and alcohol use disorders. *Current Addiction Reports, 10*(2), 122–130. https://doi.org/10.1007/s40429-023-00483-6

Koudys, J. W., Traynor, J. M., Rodrigo, A. H., Carcone, D., & Ruocco, A. C. (2019). The NIMH research domain criteria (RDoC) initiative and its implications for research on personality disorder. *Current Psychiatry Reports, 21*, 1–12. https://doi.org/10.1007/s11920-019-1023-2

Krueger, R. F., & Hobbs, K. A. (2020). An overview of the DSM-5 alternative model of personality disorders. *Psychopathology, 53*(3–4), 126–132. https://doi.org/10.1159/000508538

Krueger, R. F., Hobbs, K. A., Conway, C. C., Dick, D. M., Dretsch, M. N., Eaton, N. R., et al. (2021). Validity and utility of hierarchical taxonomy of psychopathology (HiTOP): II. Externalizing superspectrum. *World Psychiatry, 20*(2), 171–193. https://doi.org/10.1002/wps.20844

Krueger, R. F., Kotov, R., Watson, D., Forbes, M. K., Eaton, N. R., Ruggero, C. J., et al. (2018). Progress in achieving quantitative classification of psychopathology. *World Psychiatry, 17*(3), 282–293. https://doi.org/10.1002/wps.20844

Lahey, B. B., Moore, T. M., Kaczkurkin, A. N., & Zald, D. H. (2021). Hierarchical models of psychopathology: Empirical support, implications, and remaining issues. *World Psychiatry, 20*(1), 57–63. https://doi.org/10.1002/wps.20824

Landi, G., Grossman-Giron, A., Bitan, D. T., Mikulincer, M., Grandi, S., & Tossani, E. (2021). Mental pain, psychological distress, and suicidal ideation during the COVID-19 emergency: The moderating role of tolerance for mental pain. *International Journal of Mental Health and Addiction, 21*, 1–12. https://doi.org/10.1007/s11469-021-00646-4

Lind, M., Adler, J. M., & Clark, L. A. (2020). Narrative identity and personality disorder: An empirical and conceptual review. *Current Psychiatry Reports, 22*, 1–11. https://doi.org/10.1007/s11920-020-01187-8

Linhartová, P., Látalová, A., Barteček, R., Širůček, J., Theiner, P., Ejova, A., et al. (2020). Impulsivity in patients with borderline personality disorder: A comprehensive profile compared with healthy people and patients with ADHD. *Psychological Medicine, 50*(11), 1829–1838. https://doi.org/10.1017/S0033291719001892

Malhi, G. S., Das, P., Outhred, T., Bryant, R. A., & Calhoun, V. D. (2022). An fMRI examination of the neural basis of suicide attempts: The role of mentalizing in the context of mood. *Bipolar Disorders, 24*(8), 806–816. https://doi.org/10.1111/bdi.13261

Markon, K. E. (2021). On hierarchically-informed measures of psychopathology. *World Psychiatry, 20*(1), 66. https://doi.org/10.1002/wps.20812

McClelland, H., Evans, J. J., & O'Connor, R. C. (2021). Exploring the role of loneliness in relation to self-injurious thoughts and behaviour in the context of the integrated motivational-volitional model. *Journal of psychiatric research, 141*, 309–317. https://doi.org/10.1016/j.jpsychires.2021.07.020

McClelland, H., Cleare, S., & O'Connor, R. C. (2023). Suicide risk in personality disorders: A systematic review. *Current Psychiatry Reports, 25*(9), 405–417. https://doi.org/10.1007/s11920-023-01440-w

McHugh, C., & Balaratnasingam, S. (2018). Impulsivity in personality disorders: current views and future directions. *Current Opinion in Psychiatry, 31*(1), 63–68. https://doi.org/10.1097/YCO.0000000000000383

Nelson, R. K., Lass, A. N., Fanning, J. R., McCloskey, M. S., Winer, E. S., & Berman, M. E. (2022). A network model of borderline personality traits, aggression, and self-harm. *Journal of Affective Disorders Reports, 8*, 100330. https://doi.org/10.1016/j.jadr.2022.100330

Newhill, C. E., Eack, S. M., & Mulvey, E. P. (2009). Violent behavior in borderline personality. *Journal of personality disorders, 23*(6), 541–554. https://doi.org/10.1521/pedi.2009.23.6.541

Nestor, B. A., & Sutherland, S. (2022). Theory of mind and suicidality: A meta-analysis. *Archives of Suicide Research, 26*(4), 1666–1687. https://doi.org/10.1080/13811118.2021.1939209
O'Connor, R. C., & Kirtley, O. J. (2018). The integrated motivational–volitional model of suicidal behaviour. *Philosophical Transactions of the Royal Society B: Biological Sciences, 373*(1754), 20170268. https://doi.org/10.1098/rstb.2017.0268
Ordóñez-Carrasco, J. L., Cuadrado-Guirado, I., & Rojas-Tejada, A. J. (2020). Experiential avoidance in the context of the integrated motivational–volitional model of suicidal behavior. *Crisis, 42*(4), 284. https://doi.org/10.1027/0227-5910/a000721
Pearlstein, J. G., Johnson, S. L., Timpano, K. R., Stamatis, C. A., Robison, M., & Carver, C. S. (2024). Emotion-related impulsivity across transdiagnostic dimensions of psychopathology. *Journal of Personality, 92*(2), 342–360. https://doi.org/10.1111/jopy.12825
Pérez-Balaguer, A., Peñuelas-Calvo, I., Alacreu-Crespo, A., Baca-Garcia, E., & Porras-Segovia, A. (2022). Impulsivity as a mediator between childhood maltreatment and suicidal behavior: A systematic review and meta-analysis. *Journal of Psychiatric Research, 151*, 95–107. https://doi.org/10.1016/j.jpsychires.2022.04.021
Ringwald, W. R., Forbes, M. K., & Wright, A. G. (2023). Meta-analysis of structural evidence for the Hierarchical Taxonomy of Psychopathology (HiTOP) model. *Psychological Medicine, 53*(2), 533–546. https://doi.org/10.1017/S0033291721001902
Rogers, M. L., & Joiner, T. E., Jr. (2016). Borderline personality disorder diagnostic criteria as risk factors for suicidal behavior through the lens of the interpersonal theory of suicide. *Archives of Suicide Research, 20*(4), 591–604. https://doi.org/10.1080/13811118.2016.1158681
Ruggero, C. J., Kotov, R., Hopwood, C. J., First, M., Clark, L. A., Skodol, A. E., et al. (2019). Integrating the Hierarchical Taxonomy of Psychopathology (HiTOP) into clinical practice. *Journal of Consulting and Clinical Psychology, 87*(12), 1069. https://psycnet.apa.org/doi/10.1037/ccp0000452
Salsman, N. L., & Linehan, M. M. (2012). An investigation of the relationships among negative affect, difficulties in emotion regulation, and features of borderline personality disorder. *Journal of Psychopathology and Behavioral Assessment, 34*, 260–267. https://doi.org/10.1007/s10862-012-9275-8
San Too, L., Spittal, M. J., Bugeja, L., Reifels, L., Butterworth, P., & Pirkis, J. (2019). The association between mental disorders and suicide: a systematic review and meta-analysis of record linkage studies. *Journal of affective disorders, 259*, 302–313. https://doi.org/10.1016/j.jad.2019.08.054
Sastre-Buades, A., Alacreu-Crespo, A., Courtet, P., Baca-Garcia, E., & Barrigon, M. L. (2021). Decision-making in suicidal behavior: A systematic review and meta-analysis. *Neuroscience & Biobehavioral Reviews, 131*, 642–662. https://doi.org/10.1016/j.neubiorev.2021.10.005
Schreiner, M. W., Klimes-Dougan, B., Begnel, E. D., & Cullen, K. R. (2015). Conceptualizing the neurobiology of non-suicidal self-injury from the perspective of the Research Domain Criteria Project. *Neuroscience & Biobehavioral Reviews, 57*, 381–391. https://doi.org/10.1016/j.neubiorev.2015.09.011
Schuck, A., Calati, R., Barzilay, S., Bloch-Elkouby, S., & Galynker, I. (2019). Suicide Crisis Syndrome: A review of supporting evidence for a new suicide-specific diagnosis. *Behavioral Sciences & the Law, 37*(3), 223–239. https://doi.org/10.1002/bsl.2397
Sebastian, A., Jacob, G., Lieb, K., & Tüscher, O. (2013). Impulsivity in borderline personality disorder: A matter of disturbed impulse control or a facet of emotional dysregulation? *Current Psychiatry Reports, 15*, 1–8. https://doi.org/10.1007/s11920-012-0339-y
Sekowski, M., Gambin, M., Sumlin, E., & Sharp, C. (2022). Associations between symptoms of borderline personality disorder and suicidality in inpatient adolescents: The significance of identity disturbance. *Psychiatry Research, 312*, 114558. https://doi.org/10.1016/j.psychres.2022.114558
Shafti, M., Taylor, P. J., Forrester, A., & Pratt, D. (2021). The co-occurrence of self-harm and aggression: A cognitive-emotional model of dual-harm. *Frontiers in Psychology, 12*, 586135. https://doi.org/10.3389/fpsyg.2021.586135

Sharp, C., & Wall, K. (2021). DSM-5 level of personality functioning: Refocusing personality disorder on what it means to be human. *Annual Review of Clinical Psychology, 17*(1), 313–337. https://doi.org/10.1146/annurev-clinpsy-081219-105402

Sheets, E., & Craighead, W. E. (2007). Toward an empirically based classification of personality pathology. Clinical Psychology: *Science and Practice, 14*(2), 77. https://doi.org/10.1111/j.1468-2850.2007.00065.x

Sisti, D., Mann, J. J., & Oquendo, M. A. (2020). Toward a distinct mental disorder—Suicidal behavior. *JAMA Psychiatry, 77*(7), 661–662. https://doi.org/10.1001/jamapsychiatry.2020.0111

Sokol, Y., & Eisenheim, E. (2016). The relationship between continuous identity disturbances, negative mood, and suicidal ideation. *The Primary Care Companion for CNS Disorders, 18*(1), 26150. https://doi.org/10.4088/PCC.15m01824

Somma, A., Fossati, A., Ferrara, M., Fantini, F., Galosi, S., Krueger, R. F., et al. (2019). DSM-5 personality domains as correlates of non-suicidal self-injury severity in an Italian sample of adolescent inpatients with self-destructive behaviour. *Personality and Mental Health, 13*(4), 205–214. https://doi.org/10.1002/pmh.1462

Souza, K., Sosu, E. M., Thomson, S., & Rasmussen, S. (2024). A systematic review of the studies testing the integrated motivational-volitional model of suicidal behaviour. *Health Psychology Review, 18*, 1–25. https://doi.org/10.1080/17437199.2024.2336013

Steinberg, L. J., & Mann, J. J. (2020). Abnormal stress responsiveness and suicidal behavior: A risk phenotype. *Biomarkers in Neuropsychiatry, 2*, 100011. https://doi.org/10.1016/j.bionps.2020.100011

Stepp, S. D., Smith, T. D., Morse, J. Q., Hallquist, M. N., & Pilkonis, P. A. (2012). Prospective associations among borderline personality disorder symptoms, interpersonal problems, and aggressive behaviors. *Journal of Interpersonal Violence, 27*(1), 103–124. https://doi.org/10.1177/0886260511416468

Stewart, J. G., Polanco-Roman, L., Duarte, C. S., & Auerbach, R. P. (2019). Neurocognitive processes implicated in adolescent suicidal thoughts and behaviors: Applying an RDoC framework for conceptualizing risk. *Current Behavioral Neuroscience Reports, 6*, 188–196. https://doi.org/10.1007/s40473-019-00194-1

Strack, F., & Deutsch, R. (2004). Reflective and impulsive determinants of social behavior. *Personality and Social Psychology Review, 8*(3), 220–247. https://doi.org/10.1207/s15327957pspr0803_1

Taylor, P. J., McDonald, J., Smith, M., Nicholson, H., & Forrester, R. (2019). Distinguishing people with current, past, and no history of non-suicidal self-injury: Shame, social comparison, and self-concept integration. *Journal of Affective Disorders, 246*, 182–188. https://doi.org/10.1016/j.jad.2018.12.033

Terzi, L., Martino, F., Berardi, D., Bortolotti, B., Sasdelli, A., & Menchetti, M. (2017). Aggressive behavior and self-harm in Borderline Personality Disorder: The role of impulsivity and emotion dysregulation in a sample of outpatients. *Psychiatry Research, 249*, 321–326. https://doi.org/10.1016/j.psychres.2017.01.011

Tsai, M., Lari, H., Saffy, S., & Klonsky, E. D. (2021). Examining the three-step theory (3ST) of suicide in a prospective study of adult psychiatric inpatients. *Behavior Therapy, 52*(3), 673–685. https://doi.org/10.1016/j.beth.2020.08.007

Türk, N., Arslan, G., Kaya, A., Güç, E., & Turan, M. E. (2024). Psychological maltreatment, meaning-centered coping, psychological flexibility, and suicide cognitions: A moderated mediation model. *Child Abuse & Neglect, 152*, 106735. https://doi.org/10.1016/j.chiabu.2024.106735

Turner, D., Sebastian, A., & Tüscher, O. (2017). Impulsivity and cluster B personality disorders. *Current Psychiatry Reports, 19*, 1–14. https://doi.org/10.1007/s11920-017-0768-8

Turton, H., Berry, K., Danquah, A., & Pratt, D. (2021). The relationship between emotion dysregulation and suicide ideation and behaviour: A systematic review. *Journal of Affective Disorders Reports, 5*, 100136. https://doi.org/10.1016/j.jadr.2021.100136

Valenciano-Mendoza, E., Fernández-Aranda, F., Granero, R., Vintró-Alcaraz, C., Mora-Maltas, B., Valero-Solís, S., Sánchez, I., Toro, J. J., Gómez-Peña, M., Moragas, L., & Jiménez-

Murcia, S. (2022). Common and differential risk factors behind suicidal behavior in patients with impulsivity-related disorders: The case of bulimic spectrum eating disorders and gambling disorder. *Journal of Behavioral Addictions, 11*(4), 963–978. https://doi.org/10.1556/2006.2022.00072
Van Orden, K. A., Witte, T. K., Cukrowicz, K. C., Braithwaite, S. R., Selby, E. A., & Joiner Jr, T. E. (2010). The interpersonal theory of suicide. *Psychological review, 117*(2), 575. https://doi.org/10.1037/a0018697
Waller, R., Wagner, N. J., Barstead, M. G., Subar, A., Petersen, J. L., Hyde, J. S., & Hyde, L. W. (2020). A meta-analysis of the associations between callous-unemotional traits and empathy, prosociality, and guilt. *Clinical Psychology Review, 75*, 101809. https://doi.org/10.1016/j.cpr.2019.101809
Watts, A. L., Greene, A. L., Bonifay, W., & Fried, E. I. (2024). A critical evaluation of the p-factor literature. *Nature Reviews Psychology, 3*(2), 108–122. https://doi.org/10.1038/s44159-023-00260-2
Widiger, T. A., Bach, B., Chmielewski, M., Clark, L. A., DeYoung, C., Hopwood, C. J., Kotov, R., Krueger, R. F., Miller, J. D., Morey, L. C., Mullins-Sweatt, S. N., Patrick, C. J., Pincus, A. L., Samuel, D. B., Sellbom, M., South, S. C., Tackett, J. L., Watson, D., Waugh, M. H., Wright, A. G. C., et al. (2019). Criterion A of the AMPD in HiTOP. *Journal of Personality Assessment, 101*(4), 345–355. https://doi.org/10.1080/00223891.2018.1465431
Widiger, T. A., Sellbom, M., Chmielewski, M., Clark, L. A., DeYoung, C. G., Kotov, R., et al. (2019). Personality in a hierarchical model of psychopathology. *Clinical Psychological Science, 7*(1), 77–92. https://doi.org/10.1177/2167702618797105
Winsper, C., Bilgin, A., Thompson, A., Marwaha, S., Chanen, A. M., Singh, S. P., et al. (2020). The prevalence of personality disorders in the community: A global systematic review and meta-analysis. *The British Journal of Psychiatry, 216*(2), 69–78. https://doi.org/10.1192/bjp.2019.166
Yen, S., Peters, J. R., Nishar, S., Grilo, C. M., Sanislow, C. A., Shea, M. T., et al. (2021). Association of borderline personality disorder criteria with suicide attempts: Findings from the collaborative longitudinal study of personality disorders over 10 years of follow-up. *JAMA Psychiatry, 78*(2), 187–194. https://doi.org/10.1001/jamapsychiatry.2020.3598

Chapter 5
Resilience and Gender Affirmation: Coping Suicidality in Transgender and Gender Nonconforming People

Claudio Martínez, Alemka Tomicic, Angelo Brandelli Costa, Itala Raymundo Chinazzo, and Bianca Soll

5.1 Suicidality in Transgender and Gender Nonconforming People

The word transgender serves as an all-encompassing term that includes a varied spectrum of individuals who encounter a discordance between their self-perceived gender identity and the gendered society attributes to them based on their birth sex (Bockting, 2014).

The transgender and gender nonconforming (TGNC)[1] community is marginalized in many societies around the world. Discrimination and stigmatization are prevalent in these communities, limiting their access to essential social opportunities and rights. This discrimination reflects a culture of stigmatization rooted in the systemic oppression of gender minorities and the assumption of cisnormativity. This assumption holds that the norm for gender identity is to reflect the socially

[1] The authors recognize the wide variety of sexual and gender identities that exist, but in this chapter, to refer to transgender or transsexual people, the acronym TGNC refers to "trans and gender nonconforming people," or just trans* with an asterisk, which underlines the openness of what the category may contain.

C. Martínez (✉) · A. Tomicic
Faculty of Psychology, Universidad Diego Portales, Santiago, Chile

Millennium Institute for Research in Depression and Personality (MIDAP), Santiago, Chile
e-mail: claudio.martinez@mail.udp.cl

A. Brandelli Costa
Programa de Pós-Graduação em Psicologia, Pontifícia Universidade Católica do Rio Grande do Sul, Porto Alegre, Brazil

I. R. Chinazzo · B. Soll
Universidade Federal do Rio Grande do Sul, Porto Alegre, Brazil

Á. Jiménez-Molina, V. Martínez (eds.), *New Perspectives on Suicidal Behavior*, Depression and Personality, https://doi.org/10.1007/978-3-031-96037-6_5

expected form of the physical sex assigned at birth and that both sex and gender correspond to binary categories (Hughto-White et al., 2015; Martínez & Tomicic, 2023; Puckett et al., 2019; Restar & Reisner, 2017).

Discrimination and stigmatization toward TGNC people manifest themselves in various forms, such as family rejection, lack of access to adequate medical care, physical and verbal violence, and social exclusion. The chronic stress caused by these negative experiences, as well as the lack of social support, can increase the risk of developing mental health problems in TGNC people. Therefore, discrimination and stigma contribute to elevated rates of psychopathology among TGNC people, including depression and suicidal behavior. In addition, lack of access to appropriate and culturally competent mental health services can also be a barrier to obtaining needed support (Martínez et al., 2019).

Discrimination against TGNC people is not only a phenomenon limited to a particular region or country but is a global one. In many parts of the world, TGNC people face discriminatory laws and policies that limit their rights and freedoms. This can lead to social exclusion, harassment, and physical and verbal violence. Also, TGNC people may face difficulties in education, employment, and housing due to discrimination (e.g., Medina & Mahowald, 2022).

The rate of suicide attempts and self-harming behaviors is significantly higher among TGNC individuals in comparison to the general population. Specifically, concerning transgender and gender-diverse youth, the literature reports prevalence rates of suicide attempts and self-injurious behaviors between 23% and 50% higher than their cisgender peers (Coleman et al., 2022; Klein & Golub, 2016; Moody & Grant, 2013; Peterson et al., 2017; Tucker, 2019; Virupaksha et al., 2016). Furthermore, in the latest national LGBTQ youth mental health survey of 14.547 transgender and nonbinary youth who responded to the study, approximately 51% acknowledged that they had, at some point, seriously considered suicide (The Trevor Project, 2023).

Although comparisons of suicide rates between TGNC people and the general population are limited by the lack of gender identity-specific data collection in many countries, most existing studies suggest that TGNC people have higher suicide rates than the general population. For example, in studies conducted in Sweden and Australia, transgender people were found to have 19 and six times higher suicide rates than the general population, respectively. Both studies highlight the importance of addressing factors that contribute to this elevated rate of suicide and self-harming behaviors in the TGNC population, such as discrimination, lack of social support, and lack of access to health services (Dhejne et al., 2016; Zwickl et al., 2021).

This chapter will thoroughly show existing studies on suicidality within the TGNC community, concentrating specifically on the Latin American region. Subsequently, we will delve into the Minority Stress Model, highlighting its direct relevance to this group and the factors that lead to increased instances of suicidality among both young and mature TGNC individuals. Moreover, we will introduce and illustrate a comprehensive model of TGNC youth's identity formation and their experiences in dealing with suicidal thoughts and feelings. Lastly, we will provide empirical data and examine the role of gender affirmation processes (psychological, societal, and medical) in mitigating suicidal tendencies within this community and bolstering overall mental health.

5.2 The Challenges Faced by TGNC People in Latin America

In Latin America, LGBT political rights have developed and are intertwined with the achievements of social movements and the democratization of countries (Corrales & Pecheny, 2010). For more than a decade, in countries such as Uruguay, Argentina, Chile, Brazil, Colombia, Ecuador, and Bolivia, some laws allow TGNC people to change their names and gender on documents without any type of requirement, such as a medical report, or gender-affirming surgeries.

In the opposite direction, countries like Paraguay and Venezuela do not have laws related to gender identity/expression (Malta et al., 2019). However, even considering that LGBT political rights are advancing in a large part of the continent, the rates of violence and mental health vulnerabilities of this population are alarming (Henry et al., 2021; Lanham et al., 2019; Radusky et al., 2020). For example, an Argentine cross-sectional study showed that 33% of the transgender population analyzed had at least one suicide attempt throughout their lives, among whom the average age at the first attempt was adolescence (Marshall et al., 2016).

The survey *T* conducted in Chile by the Trans Diversity Organization [OTD] identified that 56.6% of the trans persons surveyed had had suicide attempts, with early adolescence (11–15 years old) being the period with the highest number of attempts (OTD, 2017). Also, in Chile, more recently, it was observed that 68% of the transgender and gender nonconforming population studied had suicidal ideation (Guzmán-González et al., 2020). In turn, a study with Brazilian transgender adults found a prevalence of 67.7% for experiencing suicidal ideation and 43.1% for having attempted suicide; among those who attempted suicide, 80.5% reported associating their attempt with being a transgender person (Chinazzo et al., 2020).

Another study carried out with binary transgender adults and *travesties* in one Brazilian state found a prevalence of 41.4% for suicidal ideation (Silva et al., 2021). In the same country, another research with transgender adults, based on the medical records of a health clinic, found a prevalence of 73.7% for suicidal ideation, and 29.9% had attempted suicide at some point in their lives. Also, the study found significant differences among young people, with a higher prevalence of 79.2% among those aged 18–20 and 88.7% among those aged 21–25 (Corrêa et al., 2020). Among Brazilian TGNC youth, a study found that 72.4% reported suicidal ideation and 42.4% suicide attempts (Chinazzo et al., 2023). The studies above also found an association between the presence of suicidal ideation and suicide attempts and discrimination experiences; on the contrary, receiving social support was associated with lower rates of both outcomes (Chinazzo et al., 2020, 2023).

Additionally, although these data revealed the need for mental health services for TGNC people in general and the younger ones, many countries in Latin America have also encountered problems in implementing health policies aimed at the transgender population, which would end up implying a failure in the implementation of their rights. Brazil is an example of this; despite the legal rights and the healthcare gender affirmation being public, TGNC people have difficulty accessing these services due to discrimination, lack of information, and a policy design that does not meet the needs of the population and can take an average of 9 years (Costa et al., 2018; Soll et al., 2017).

5.3 Minority Stress Model and Disparities in Suicidality in the TGNC Population

The Minority Stress Model (Meyer, 2003) is one of the most essential and valuable theories for understanding how the social processes of discrimination underlie negative mental health indicators in sexual and gender minority populations. This model identifies processes that constitute sources of stress for minorities and that can be classified as distal (i.e., contextual and structural) or proximal (i.e., individual and subjective) (Meyer, 2007). Minority stress is distinguished from general stress by its origin in prejudice and stigma. Thus, a stressor, such as being insulted in the street, could be a general stressor or a minority stressor depending on whether it is motivated by prejudice against a person belonging to a sexual and gender minority, as opposed to, for example, a traffic discussion that could affect all people regardless of their sexual and gender identity (Frost & Meyer, 2023).

This model was initially developed specifically with cisgender sexual minorities—that is, lesbians, gays, and bisexuals—but in recent years has been empirically applied to the TGNC people, showing its potential for understanding the effect of the negative and challenging experiences that they face (Scandurra et al., 2017a, 2017b; Tan et al., 2020). Conjunctly, these studies roughly demonstrate that experiencing violence and discrimination at high rates leads TGNC people to direct negative social attitudes toward themselves while resisting and counteracting the stigma installed in a society that discriminates based on gender identity (Testa et al., 2015). As some authors have suggested, this stigma affects the mental health of TGNC people at structural, interpersonal, and individual levels. Each of these dimensions has been studied separately, but there has been a progressive increase in studies that seek to assess how they interact and overlap (Hughto et al., 2015; Reisner et al., 2016; Scandurra et al., 2018).

It appears that in the interplay between these three dimensions, the stressor most strongly associated with mental health problems and suicidality is internalized stigma, that is, concern about one's own identity due to internalization of the gender expectations and norms of the society in which one develops, which may be directed against oneself (vertical internalized transphobia) and against other TGNC people (horizontal internalized transphobia) (Coleman et al., 2022). Internalized stigma in TGNC youth may exacerbate clinically significant symptoms of posttraumatic stress disorder, suicidal thoughts, or nonsuicidal self-injury (Reisner et al., 2016; Taliaferro et al., 2018; Wilson & Liss, 2022). Some authors have emphasized that this stigma "gets under the skin" (Hatzenbuehler, 2009) and participates as a mediator in psychological processes that affect emotional regulation as well as in interpersonal conflicts and cognitive processes that carry a risk of psychopathology. Examples of this include the psychological mediator role played by daily rumination on aspects associated with stigma and victimization in the impact on depression and suicidality in TGNC individuals (Puckett et al., 2023; Sarno et al., 2020).

5.4 Identity Development and Suicidal Processes

From a comprehensive perspective that has sought to delve into the subjective experience of suicidality in TGNC people, it has been possible to establish specific common patterns in young people that allow us to look at the interaction between moments of adolescent development with the social emergence of trans* identity.

In a study that analyzed the subjective construction that a group of eight Chilean trans youth made of their experience of having lived through and survived a suicidal process, it appeared that this experience was intertwined with aspects of the process of emergence of trans identity (Martínez et al., 2024). In this process, the study identified three moments associated with identity development that appear to be related to different recognizable risk factors in a suicide process. The first moment that we call *questioning, confusion, and exploration of the transgender identity* is characterized by a feeling of alienation and an altered emotional state, in which the fear of losing significant relationships becomes particularly intense. A second moment called *beginning to understand* one's own transgender identity is characterized by anxiety and fear in anticipation of the difficulties of daily life that place them in a permanent survival mode.

In the following fragment, a transgender woman accounts for the passage from the first moment of questioning, confusion, and exploration to the second one of beginning to understand, mentioning some of the risk factors of suicide in her experience:

> Since I started to realize I was a transgender woman, since then things no longer were..., before I thought, well... what I think and feel maybe it is just clothes or wanting to look like [a woman], (...) I slowly realized and I thought 'well what I have to do is something, but it is the hardest part' so since then I sometimes thought about how I could do this, that I was going to be left alone, that I could lose my career, my family, everyone (...) so I remember when I was younger I often thought about it [suicide] but I never... I never said I was going to do it now—it was just an idea; I wish that would happen to me, I wish I did not wake up tomorrow—stuff like that" (Martínez et al., 2024).

As can be seen, the fear of losing significant others because of her identity and the anticipation of a challenging daily life appear as too-specific risk factors of suicide intertwined with the process of gender identity development. Finally, the third moment, being trans*, is characterized by the question of how to exist with a transgender identity, whose response can be ambivalent between freezing panic with a mood of hopelessness and, on the other hand, beginning to make decisions regarding the diverse ways of existing in the world through the transition of their identity. In the following excerpt, a transgender man explains this ambivalent position and suggests that its resolution has to do with quitting his very precious dream:

> I: What was your question? Will I be transgender, or do I want to be a man or not?
>
> R: If I want to or not, because inside I know I want to, but the problem is everything that is required to achieve that; everything about the transition is difficult for me, so the possibility goes down, then I have hope (…), and then I do not know (…). Yeah, and that makes me even more confused, like, 'Do I really not want this, or is it because it is very complicated?' So, then I know that I want it, but as time goes by, I am thinking about if I will be able, so I get discouraged, in a way, and I leave it aside like in a dream I cannot reach, so that is why I… (Martínez et al., 2024).

These three moments do not occur linearly and may show back-and-forth movements, implying deep feelings of hopelessness. Also, they are represented in the interviewees' references to their lives as trans young people facing an uncertain future where the primary source of hopelessness has to do with their doubts about their right to exist, which slowly invades them as they begin to understand their identity. This issue is compounded by various social barriers that are believed to accelerate suicidal processes.

In the process described above, the role of the family is fundamental. The conviction that being trans is "weird" and may harm loved ones, especially parents, certainly forces them to question their existence (Cardona et al., 2021; Clark et al., 2022). Typically, the family is an arena in which doubts about one's right to exist as a trans person can deepen, whether fantasized or real; family rejection or acceptance is a significant source of this uncertainty. In this regard, Ryan et al. (2010) demonstrated that young trans adults who had experienced high levels of family rejection were more likely to experience depression and attempted suicide during adolescence than those who had not been rejected. In contrast, when there is a supportive and loving family, state, and culture that recognizes gender identity (e.g., social name use), trans* people would be expected to be less likely to die by suicide (Green et al., 2021).

On the other hand, when young people achieve by telling their stories a subjective position that highlights hope, survival, and what some authors have called resilience in minority groups (Frost & Meyer, 2012), in addition to reflecting on their suicidal process, allow them to identify elements that helped them to survive (Martínez et al., 2024). For example, some highlight the relevance of identifying with trans* media figures, allowing them to find protection and expectations of existence by constructing a positive and forward-looking identity (Liu et al., 2021). Resilience is often operationalized as individual-level attributes and community-level resources external to the individual (Frost & Meyer, 2009). In this sense, Individual aspects of resilience may emerge in individual processes of psychotherapeutic accompaniment.

In this regard, Meyer (2015) highlights the role of community engagement, not only because it appears to have a transformative effect on individuals but also because it strengthens the community itself, known as community connectedness. In research, Chodzen et al. (2019) found that trans youth's lack of connectivity with their communities was associated with higher indicators of depression in them.

Another identity aspect that, at some moments of development, interacts intensely with suicidality is the bodily dimension of trans people. From the first manifestations that mark the beginning of a person's doubts during puberty to their frustrations associated with eroticization and the possibilities of love, all of them are informed by the daily presence of what has been called the "mirror trauma" (Langer, 2016; Martínez et al., 2024). Few studies have explored the connection between trans people's subjective bodily experience and their mental health. The literature generally references an incongruent biological and anatomical body that may be aligned with or confirmed by individual identity (Bockting, 2014). Nevertheless, the body is an essential element for trans* people, as it is the form through which gender is manifested in our culture.

Therefore, for young trans people, bodily development accompanies their identity, not only through its effect on their interactions with the world but also through the internal sensations that shape bodily awareness (Langer, 2019). In this context, it has been pointed out that trans people suffer a double trauma: gender trauma due to discordance and incongruence and everyday trauma due to rejection, discrimination, and violence (Langer, 2019). Thus, it is not difficult to understand how the cumulative weight of this dual trauma can affect mental health, ultimately leading to suicidal ideation or suicide attempts.

5.5 Gender Affirmation and Other Protective Factors

Studies emphasizing interactions between individual and social factors have highlighted the need to look at the multiplicity of biological, interpersonal, social, and contextual variables that surround mental health risks for TGNC individuals (Reisner et al., 2016). To mitigate those risks and build resilience, there is a need for a comprehensive approach that includes an affirmation of gender diversity as a critical aspect of public health, healthcare based on quality evidence, and effective alliances with local trans* communities to ensure responsiveness and cultural specificity in intervention planning (Snow et al., 2019).

Therefore, gender affirmation is a critical social determinant in the health of TGNC people (Bockting, 2014). It has been defined as an interpersonal and shared process through which a person's gender identity is socially recognized, which in turn involves aspects of health and the legal order of the cultural and social context in which this process unfolds (Nuttbrock et al., 2009; Sevelius, 2013).

As one would expect, gender affirmation involves various factors, such as the social and legal context, accessibility to hormone treatment, culturally competent healthcare providers, and psychological aspects, such as the recognition and the work on the internalized stigma (Bockting, 2008). There is no single path to gender affirmation since it comes to fruition in temporal trajectories that are not necessarily linear or consecutive, and in which, according to Kuper et al. (2018), the following moments or milestones can be identified: (1) awareness of nonconformity or disagreement with the assigned gender; (2) the exploration of aspects of a gender different from the one assigned; (3) the creation of a sense of identity different from cisgender heteronormativity; and (4) the process of integrating experiences of gender discordance and concordance into a global sense of self.

Regarding the consequences of his psychotherapeutic process, a transgender male states that self-awareness has been one of the most important outcomes of his affirmative process:

> ...And, I do not know, like the most important thing, of course, is to generate this own sense of security and along the way, realizing that one can resolve that as well, of untangling this whole thread of entanglement, experiences, fears, insecurities, life experiences that one carries... seeing them from a different perspective... And being more loving towards the process of change because many times, of course, one gets anxious and thinks like, damn, I do not know, "Why don't I wake up tomorrow with a face full of hair?" Like, "How do I manage the anxiety?"... so that these things do not affect me daily or that I do not have to compare myself to other people and their processes. It feels like a journey, at least for me, and it has been and is the most important thing: a journey of self-awareness. And that is what I have left and what has also led me to have this sense of security to say, "Okay, right now I do feel good," so I can tell myself, "Okay, I can give myself a break and rest a bit." (Tomicic et al., 2024).

In this context, concrete "affirmative interventions" refer to those that promote the congruence of the experience of gender identity with legal, social, and corporal dimensions (Coleman et al., 2022; Kuper et al., 2018). The evidence indicates that these interventions promote general well-being in trans* people (Coleman et al., 2022; Sevelius et al., 2021). For example, a decrease in anxious and depressive symptoms and an increase in social, psychological, and sexual well-being have been reported after affirmative medical interventions such as surgery or hormonal treatment (Agarwal et al., 2018; Owen-Smith et al., 2018; Davis & Meier, 2014). Concerning the impacts of body affirmation on well-being, in the following fragment, a transgender man illustrates this from his experience with the first results of hormone therapy:

> It is going to sound funny, but I have a crazy little hair here on my beard [chin], haha, but it is like a crazy little hair, literally.
>
> I: But is it like you check yourself?
>
> Yes, in the beginning, you look at yourself all the time, I do not know what, the back and consistently. You start to relax, and it is like, out of nowhere… ooh, look, I have a mustache and many mustaches. However, the first few times, you keep looking in the mirror, waiting for the change, but it comes as soon as you lose focus. However, that excited me a lot, and when my back got more expansive, it was super exciting and annoying" (Martínez et al. (2023/2027)).

In a recent review of the literature on the role of medical affirmation treatments (hormones, puberty blockers, and surgery) in reducing suicidality in TGNC individuals, it was found that in most of the research reviewed, there was a reduction in the level of suicidality of individuals. Still, the author emphasized the importance of keeping in mind the methodological limitations of most of the studies; effect size, history of psychiatric treatment, comorbidity with substance use, the interaction of time elapsed since receiving gender-affirming treatment, and others were elements that were unclear or not sufficiently controlled for (Jackson, 2023). While this does not diminish the positive effect reported mainly by studies on gender-affirming treatments (Coleman et al., 2022; Sevelius et al., 2021), it does raise a red flag for the need to improve the methodology that primarily uses suicidality as an indicator (Marques et al., 2023).

5.6 Mental Health Interventions with Trans Populations

As mentioned before, in the Minority Stress Model (Meyer, 2003), internalized sexual stigma refers to the internalization of prejudice and discriminatory attitudes of individuals belonging to a sexual and gender minority as part of their value system, adapting and conforming to social stigmatization.

The Psychological Mediation Framework, or PMF (Hatzenbuehler, 2009), an extension of the Minority Stress Theory, incorporates a more clinical and nuanced view of minority stress, recognizing that stressors do not have the same impact on all individuals. This framework sheds light on how stigma-related chronic stressors might lead to adverse mental health outcomes if distal stressors (e.g., discrimination) affect mental health through the mediating action of proximal stressors (e.g., internalized transphobia). Resilience factors can also play a crucial role in the relationship between minority stress and mental health by mitigating the detrimental effects of stress and stigma (Freese et al., 2018; Meyer, 2015; Puckett et al., 2020).

Among these resilience factors are personal qualities that individuals can use to effectively ameliorate the detrimental effect of stressors on health, such as pride in one's trans* identity (Bockting et al., 2013). For example, TGNC people who "mentalize stigma" (i.e., who can understand their reactions to stigmatizing and discriminatory experiences, as well as the violence of others associated with stigma) are better able to mitigate the adverse effects that these experiences can have on their mental health. This means that this ability to reflect, which fosters resilience, can be a protective factor against the effects of minority stress, including suicidality (Scandurra et al., 2020).

On the other hand, authors such as Matsuno and Israel (2018) suggest using psychological interventions to strengthen other resilience factors of TGNC people, present at the community, group, and individual levels. It is noted that these psychological and psychotherapeutic interventions must be framed in an affirmative practice, approaching clinical work from a nonpathologizing position that accepts and validates gender diversity (APA, 2015; Scandurra et al., 2019). Likewise, studies that have established loneliness in trans youth as a significant mediator between internalized stigma and psychological well-being have proposed clinical interventions that stimulate social support (Garro et al., 2022). Isolation from one's community increases internalized stigma, as it generates the perception of being rejected by everyone, which, in turn, increases feelings of loneliness, depression, and easily suicidal thoughts (Inderbinen et al., 2021; Scandurra et al., 2018).

During the therapeutic process, by exploring the manifestations of internalized stigma in TGNC patients (low self-esteem, guilt, shame, etc.), the clinician can share with their patient some hypotheses associated with the Minority Stress Model (Proujansky & Panchankis, 2014). For some people, this will make sense in their histories of discrimination, and they will be able to understand some symptoms or protective strategies of avoidance, concealment, and pseudo-adaptation. For others, however, it will be more challenging to accept that some things that happen to them respond to the conceptualization of this model, instead clinging to beliefs or factors such as genetics, neurological problems, childhood traumas, or personality disorders (Martínez et al., 2018).

Once the internalized stigma has been established as the focus of therapeutic work, the next step is the development of a progressive awareness of the links between the origin of their beliefs and their negative feelings about themselves (Szymanski et al., 2014). This can empower the patient, transforming their subjective position as a victim into one in which they can influence others and participate in their community, which in turn leads them to be less isolated and, therefore, enter a virtuous circle of personal growth (Kashubeck-West et al., 2008; Martínez & Tomicic, 2023).

However, as a counterpart, TGNC individuals also face additional stigmas that intersect and often deepen internalized sexual stigma. This occurs primarily when their life trajectories have led them to marginalization from the healthcare system, education, housing, and economic support structures (Holt et al., 2020). In such cases, individuals face additional disparities in accessing healthcare services, experiencing substantial barriers to care (James et al., 2016). Therefore, affirmative mental health interventions, in addition to considering the presence of individual aspects, must also address the various social and structural determinants that act as stressors and risk factors for suicidality.

5.7 Resilience and Gender Affirmation

The issues surrounding transgender and gender nonconforming (TGNC) individuals are multifaceted and deeply rooted in societal norms and structures. Throughout this chapter, we have explored the challenges faced by the TGNC community, especially young trans* people, ranging from discrimination and stigmatization to disparities in mental health outcomes, especially high rates of suicidality. The pervasive nature of these challenges underscores the urgent need for comprehensive understanding and effective interventions.

The Minority Stress Model and Psychological Mediation Framework provide valuable frameworks for comprehending the complexities of minority stress and its impact on mental health outcomes among TGNC youth. These models highlight the interplay between external stressors, such as discrimination and internalized stigma, shedding light on the pathways through which these stressors contribute to mental health problems and suicidality.

Furthermore, the intersectionality of identity development, particularly during adolescence, adds another layer of complexity to the experiences of TGNC individuals. The concept of intersectionality to which we refer alludes to how various categories of identity, such as gender, race, social class, sexual orientation, disability, among others, intertwine and interdependently affect people's experiences of oppression and inequalities (Cho et al., 2013). For example, in Chile, the social class position is an aspect that can determine the development of an adolescent concerning his or her gender identity through the relationship with the parent's educational level, the place where he or she lives, and access to education and health.

Bear in mind the above considerations; the process of understanding and affirming transgender identity is intertwined with multiple risk factors for suicidality, including family rejection and societal barriers. However, resilience factors, such as community support and gender affirmation, can mitigate these risks and foster positive mental health outcomes. Moving forward, it is essential to adopt a holistic approach to mental health interventions for TGNC young people. Affirmative practices that validate gender diversity and address both individual and structural determinants of mental health are paramount. Additionally, psychotherapeutic interventions should empower individuals to challenge internalized stigma and cultivate resilience in adversity.

Addressing the disparities in mental health outcomes among TGNC individuals requires concerted efforts at multiple levels, including policy changes, healthcare reforms, and community support initiatives. By recognizing the unique challenges faced by the TGNC community and implementing evidence-based interventions, we can strive toward creating a more inclusive, supportive, and affirmative environment for all individuals, regardless of gender identity.

Acknowledgments This manuscript was supported by ANID—Millennium Science Initiative Program—AIM23_0002 and by ANID—Fondecyt Project N° 1230262.

References

Agarwal, C. A., Scheefer, M. F., Wright, L. N., Walzer, N. K., & Rivera, A. (2018). Quality of life improvement after chest wall masculinization in female-to-male transgender patients: A prospective study using the BREAST-Q and Body Uneasiness Test. *Journal of Plastic, Reconstructive & Aesthetic Surgery, 71*(5), 651–657. https://doi.org/10.1016/j.bjps.2018.01.003

American Psychological Association [APA]. (2015). Guidelines for psychological practice with transgender and gender nonconforming people. *American Psychologist, 70*(9), 832–864. https://doi.org/10.1037/a0039906

Bockting, W., Miner, M. H., Swinburne, R., Hamilton, A., & Coleman, E. (2013). Stigma, mental health, and resilience in an online sample of the US transgender population. *The American Journal of Public Health, 103*, 943–951. https://doi.org/10.2105/AJPH.2013.301241

Bockting, W. (2014). Transgender identity development. In D. Tolman, L. Diamond, J. Bauermeister, W. George, J. Pfaus, & M. Ward (Eds.), *APA handbook of sexuality and psychology* (pp. 739–758). American Psychological Association.

Bockting, W. (2008). Psychotherapy and the real-life experience: From gender dichotomy to gender diversity. *Sexologie, 17*, 211–224. https://doi.org/10.1016/j.sexol.2008.08.001

Cardona, N. D., Madigan, R. J., & Sauer-Zavala, S. (2021). How minority stress becomes traumatic invalidation: An emotion-focused conceptualization of minority stress in sexual and gender minority people. *Clinical Psychologist: Science and Practice*. Advance online publication. https://doi.org/10.1037/cps0000054

Chinazzo, I. R., Lobato, M. I. R., Nardi, H. C., Koller, S. H., Saadeh, A., & Costa, A. B. (2020). Impact of minority stress in depressive symptoms, suicide idea and suicide attempt in trans people. *Ciência & Saúde Coletiva, 26*(3), 5045–5056. https://doi.org/10.1590/1413-812320212611.3.28532019

Chinazzo, Í. R., Fontanari, A. M. V., Costa, A. B., & Lobato, M. I. R. (2023). Factors associated with suicidal ideation and suicide attempt in Brazilian transgender youth. *International Journal of Environmental Research and Public Health, 20*(4), 3215.

Clark, K., Salway, T., McConocha, E. M., & Pachankis, J. E. (2022). How do sexual and gender minority people acquire the capability for suicide? Voices from survivors of near-fatal suicide attempts. *SSM - Qualitative Research in Health*. https://doi.org/10.1016/j.ssmqr.2022.100044

Chodzen, G., Hidalgo, M. A., Chen, D., & Garofalo, R. (2019). Minority stress factors associated with depression and anxiety among transgender and gender-nonconforming youth. *Journal of Adolescence Health, 64*(4), 467–471. https://doi.org/10.1016/j.jadohealth.2018.07.006

Cho, S., Crenshaw, K. W., & McCall, L. (2013). Intersectionality: Theorizing power, empowering theory. *Signs, 38*(4), 785–810. https://doi.org/10.1086/669608

Coleman, E., Radix, A. E., Bouman, W. P., Brown, G. R., de Vries, A., Deutsch, M. B., Ettner, R., Fraser, L., Goodman, M., Green, J., Hancock, A. B., Johnson, T. W., Karasic, D. H., Knudson, G. A., Leibowitz, S. F., Meyer-Bahlburg, H. F. L., Monstrey, S. J., Motmans, J., Nahata, L., Nieder, T. O., et al. (2022). Standards of care for the health of transgender and gender diverse people, version 8. *International Journal of Transgender Health, 6*(23), S1–S259. https://doi.org/10.1080/26895269.2022.2100644

Corrales, J., & Pecheny, M. (Eds.). (2010). *The politics of sexuality in Latin America: A reader on lesbian, gay, bisexual, and transgender rights*. University of Pittsburgh Press. https://doi.org/10.2307/j.ctt5vkfk6

Corrêa, F. H. M., Rodrigues, B. B., Mendonça, J. C., & Cruz, L. R. D. (2020). Pensamento suicida entre a população transgênero: Um estudo epidemiológico. *Jornal Brasileiro de Psiquiatria, 69*(1), 13–22. https://doi.org/10.1590/0047-2085000000256

Costa, A. B., da Rosa Filho, H. T., Pase, P. F., Fontanari, A. M. V., Catelan, R. F., Mueller, A., Cardoso, D., Soll, B., Schwarz, K., Schneider, M. A., Gagliotti, D. A. M., Saadeh, A., Lobato, M. I. R., Nardi, H. C., & Koller, S. H. (2018). Healthcare needs of and access barriers for Brazilian transgender and gender diverse people. *Journal of Immigrant and Minority Health, 20*(1), 115–123. https://doi.org/10.1007/s10903-016-0527-7

Davis, S. A., & Meier, S. (2014). Effects of testosterone treatment and chest reconstruction surgery on mental health and sexuality in female-to-male transgender people. *International Journal of Sexual Health, 26*(2), 113–128. https://doi.org/10.1080/19317611.2013.833152

Dhejne, C., Van Vlerken, R., Heylens, G., & Arcelus, J. (2016). Mental health and gender dysphoria: A review of the literature. *International Review of Psychiatry, 28*(1), 44–57. https://doi.org/10.3109/09540261.2015.1115753

Freese, R., Ott, M. Q., Rood, B. A., Reisner, S. L., & Pantalone, D. W. (2018). Distinct coping profiles are associated with mental health differences in transgender and gender nonconforming adults. *Journal of Clinical Psychology, 74*(1), 136–146. https://doi.org/10.1002/jclp.22490

Frost, D. M., & Meyer, I. H. (2009). Internalized homophobia and relationship quality among lesbians, gay men, and bisexuals. *Journal of Counseling Psychology, 59*, 97–109. https://doi.org/10.1037/a0012844

Frost, D. M., & Meyer, I. H. (2012). Measuring community connectedness among diverse sexual minority populations. *Journal of Sex Research, 49*, 36–49. https://doi.org/10.1080/00224499.2011.565427

Frost, D. M., & Meyer, I. H. (2023). Minority stress theory: Application, critique, and continued relevance. *Current Opinion in Psychology, 51*, 101579. https://doi.org/10.1016/j.copsyc.2023.101579

Garro, M., Novara, C., Di Napoli, G., Scandurra, C., Bochicchio, V., & Lavanco, G. (2022). The role of internalized transphobia, loneliness, and social support in the psychological well-being of a group of Italian transgender and gender non-conforming youths. *Healthcare (Basel), 10*(11), 2282. https://doi.org/10.3390/healthcare10112282

Green, A. E., DeChants, J. P., Price, M. N., & Davis, C. K. (2021). Association of gender-affirming hormone therapy with depression, thoughts of suicide, and attempted suicide among transgender and nonbinary youth. *Journal of Adolescent Health, 70*(4), 643–649. https://doi.org/10.1016/j.jadohealth.2021.10.036

Guzmán-González, M., Barrientos, J., Saiz, J. L., Gómez, F., Cárdenas, M., Espinoza-Tapia, R., Bahamondes, J., Lovera, L., & Giami, A. (2020). Salud mental en población transgénero y género no conforme en Chile. *Revista Médica de Chile, 148*(8), 1113–1120. https://doi.org/10.4067/S0034-98872020000801113

Hatzenbuehler, M. L. (2009). How does sexual minority stigma "get under the skin"? A psychological mediation framework. *Psychological Bulletin, 135*(5), 707–730. https://doi.org/10.1037/a0016441

Henry, R. S., Hoetger, C., Rabinovitch, A. E., Aguayo Arelis, A., Rabago Barajas, B. V., & Perrin, P. B. (2021). Discrimination, mental health, and suicidal ideation among sexual minority adults in Latin America: Considering the roles of social support and religiosity. *Trauma Care, 1*, 143–161. https://doi.org/10.3390/traumacare1030013

Holt, N., Hope, D., Mocarski, R., Meyer, H., King, R., & Woodruff, N. (2020). The provider perspective on behavioral health care for transgender and gender nonconforming individuals in the Central Great Plains: A qualitative study of approaches and needs. *American Journal of Orthopsychiatry, 90*(1), 136–146. https://doi.org/10.1037/ort0000406

Hughto-White, J. M., Reisner, S. L., & Pachankis, J. E. (2015). Transgender stigma and health: A critical review of stigma determinants, mechanisms and interventions. *Social Science & Medicine, 147*, 222–231. https://doi.org/10.1016/j.socscimed.2015.11.010

Inderbinen, M., Schaefer, K., Schneeberger, A., Gaab, J., & Garcia, N. D. (2021). Relationship of internalized transnegativity and protective factors with depression, anxiety, non-suicidal self-injury and suicidal tendency in trans populations: A systematic review. *Frontiers in Psychiatry, 20*, 636513. https://doi.org/10.3389/fpsyt.2021.636513

Jackson, D. (2023). Suicide-related outcomes following gender-affirming treatment: A review. *Cureus, 15*(3), e36425. https://doi.org/10.7759/cureus.36425

James, S., Herman, J., Rankin, S., Keisling, M., Mottet, L., & Anafi, M. (2016). *The report of the 2015 U.S. transgender survey*. National Center for Transgender Equality.

Kashubeck-West, S., Szymanski, D., & Meyer, J. (2008). Internalized heterosexism: Clinical implications and training considerations. *The Counseling Psychologist, 36*(4), 615–630. https://doi.org/10.1177/0011000007309634

Klein, A., & Golub, S. A. (2016). Family rejection as a predictor of suicide attempts and substance misuse among transgender and gender nonconforming adults. *LGBT Health, 3*(3), 193–199. https://doi.org/10.1089/lgbt.2015.0111

Kuper, E. L., Wright, L., & Mustanski, B. (2018). Gender identity development among transgender and gender nonconforming emerging adults: An intersectional approach. *International Journal of Transgenderism, 19*(4), 436–455. https://doi.org/10.1080/15532739.2018.1443869

Langer, S. J. (2016). Trans bodies and the failure of mirrors. *Studies in Gender and Sexuality, 17*(4), 306–316. https://doi.org/10.1080/15240657.2016.1236553

Langer, S. J. (2019). *Theorizing transgender identity for clinical practice. A new model for understanding gender*. Jessica Kingsley Publisher.

Lanham, M., Ridgeway, K., Dayton, R., Castillo, B. M., Brennan, C., Davis, D. A., Emmanuel, D., Morales, G. J., Cheririser, C., Rodriguez, B., Cooke, J., Santi, K., & Evens, E. (2019). "We're Going to Leave You for Last, Because of How You Are": Transgender women's experiences of gender-based violence in healthcare, education, and police encounters in Latin America and the Caribbean. *Violence and Gender, 6*(1), 37–46. https://doi.org/10.1089/vio.2018.0015

Liu, Y., Jiang, Z., She, H., & Zhang, Y. (2021). The impact of role models on self-identity of LGBTQ teenagers. *Proceedings of the 2021 4th International Conference on Humanities Education and Social Sciences (ICHESS 2021)*. https://doi.org/10.2991/assehr.k.211220.095

Malta, M., Cardoso, R., Montenegro, L., de Jesus, J., Seixas, M., Benevides, B., das Dores Silva, M., LeGrand, S., & Whetten, K. (2019). Sexual and gender minorities rights in Latin America and the Caribbean: A multi-country evaluation. *BMC International Health and Human Rights, 19*(31). https://doi.org/10.1186/s12914-019-0217-3

Marques, I., Cagigal, C., Ezzeddine, R., Rema, J., & Cruz, F. (2023). The impact of gender-affirming surgeries on suicide-related outcomes: A systematic review. *Journal of Psychosexual Health, 5*(3), 134–144. https://doi.org/10.1177/26318318231189836

Marshall, B., Socías, M., Kerr, T., Zalazar, V., Sued, O., & Arístegui, I. (2016). Prevalence and correlates of lifetime suicide attempts among transgender persons in Argentina. *Journal of Homosexuality, 63*(7), 955–967. https://doi.org/10.1080/00918369.2015.1117898

Martinez, C., & Tomicic, A. (2023). Psychotherapy and Affirmative Practices with trans and gender non-conforming (TGNC) patients in Chile (Chapter 2). In R. Chaparro & R. Abreu (Eds.), *LGBTQ+ affirmative psychological interventions. A Latine/x perspective* (pp. 11–35). Springer.

Martínez, C., Gaete, M.I., Paiva, I., Tomicic, A., Concha, F. (2023/2027). El cuerpo soñado: estudio sobre la experiencia corporal de personas Trans* y de género no conforme (TGNC). Proyecto Fondecyt Regular 2023, ANID, Chile.

Martínez, C., Tomicic, A., & del Pino, S. (2019). Disparidades y barreras de acceso a la salud mental en personas LGBTI+: El derecho a una atención culturalmente competente [Disparities and barriers to mental health access for LGBTI+ people: The right to culturally competent care]. In F. Vargas (Ed.), *Informe Anual sobre Derechos Humanos en Chile 2019 [Annual Report on the Situation of Human Rights in Chile]*. Centro de Derechos Humanos, Universidad Diego Portales. Ediciones UDP.

Martínez, C., Tomicic, A., Gálvez, C., Rodríguez, J., Rosenbaum, C., & Aguayo, F. (2018). *Psicoterapia Culturalmente Competente para el Trabajo con Pacientes LGBT+: Una Guía para Psicoterapeutas y Profesionales de la Salud Mental [Culturally competent psychotherapy for working with LGBT+ Patients: A guide for psychotherapists and mental health professionals]*. Centro de Estudios en Psicología Clínica y Psicoterapia (CEPPS), Facultad de Psicología, Universidad Diego Portales, Santiago de Chile.

Martínez, C., Tomicic, A., Rodríguez, J., Rosenbaum, C., Aguayo, F., & Gálvez, C. (2024). Our Daily Trauma: Subjective construction about suicidal processes of trans* youth. *Psykhe, 34*(1), 1–14. https://doi.org/10.7764/psykhe.2024.81556.

Martínez, C., Gaete, M. I., Concha, F., Paiva, I., & Tomicic, A. (2023–2027). *Proyecto Fondecyt: El cuerpo soñado: estudio sobre la experiencia corporal de personas Trans* y de género no conforme (TGNC) [Fondecyt Project: The Dreamed Body: Study on the Bodily Experience of Trans* and Gender Non-Conforming (TGNC) People]*. Proyecto Fondecyt Regular 1230262. ANID, Chile.

Matsuno, E., & Israel, T. (2018). Psychological interventions promoting resilience among transgender individuals: Transgender Resilience Intervention Model (TRIM). *The Counseling Psychologist, 46*(5), 632–655. https://doi.org/10.1177/0011000018787261

Medina, C., & Mahowald, L. (2022). *Discrimination and barriers to well-being: The State of the LGBTQI+ Community in 2022*. Center for American Progress. https://www.americanprogress.org/article/discrimination-and-barriers-to-well-being-the-state-of-the-lgbtqi-community-in-2022/

Meyer, I. (2003). Prejudice, social stress and mental health in lesbian, gay and bisexual population: Conceptual issues and research evidence. *Psychological Bulletin, 129*(5), 674–697. https://doi.org/10.1037/0033-2909.129.5.674

Meyer, I. H. (2007). Prejudice and discrimination as social stressors. In I. Meyer & M. Northridge (Eds.), *The health of sexual minorities: Public health perspectives on lesbian, gay, bisexual and transgender populations* (pp. 242–267). Springer.

Meyer, I. H. (2015). Resilience in the study of minority stress and health of sexual and gender minorities. *Psychology of Sexual Orientation and Gender Diversity, 2*, 209–213. https://doi.org/10.1037/sgd0000132

Moody, C., & Grant, N. (2013). Suicide protective factors among trans adults. *Archives of Sexual Behavior, 42*, 739–752. https://doi.org/10.1007/s10508-013-0099-8

Nuttbrock, L., Bockting, W. O., Hwahng, S., Rosemblum, A., Mason, M., Macri, M., & Becker, J. (2009). Gender identity affirmation among male-to-female transgender persons: A life course analysis across types of relationships and cultural/lifestyle factors. *Sex Relationship Therapy, 24*, 108–125. https://doi.org/10.1080/14681990902926764

Organizando Trans Diversidades. (2017). *Informe sobre Encuesta T: 1era Encuesta para personas trans y de género no-conforme en Chile. Resumen ejecutivo [Report on Survey T: 1st Survey for trans and gender non-conforming people in Chile. Executive summary]*. Santiago, Chile. Disponible en: http://decs.pjud.cl/documentos/descargas/Informe_ejecutivo_Encuesta-T.pdf

Owen-Smith, A. A., Gerth, J., Sineath, R. C., Barzilay, J., Becerra-Culqui, T. A., Getahun, D., Giammattei, S., Hunkeler, E., Lash, T., Millman, A., Nash, R., Qiunn, V., Robinson, B., Roblin, D., Sanchez, T., Silverberg, M., Tangpricha, V., Valentine, C., Winterm, S., Woodyatt, C., Song, Y., & Goodman, M. (2018). Association between gender confirmation treatments and perceived gender congruence, body image satisfaction, and mental health in a cohort of transgender individuals. *The Journal of Sexual Medicine, 15*(4), 591–600. https://doi.org/10.1016/j.jsxm.2018.01.017

Peterson, C., Matthews, A., Copps-Smith, E., & Conard, L. A. (2017). Suicidality, self-harm, and body dissatisfaction in transgender adolescents and emerging adults with gender dysphoria. *Suicide and Life-Threatening Behavior, 47*(4), 475–482. https://doi.org/10.1111/sltb.12289

Proujansky, R. A., & Pachankis, J. E. (2014). Toward formulating evidence-based principles of LGB-affirmative psychotherapy. *Pragmatic Case Studies in Psychotherapy, 10*(2), 117–131. https://doi.org/10.14713/pcsp.v10i2.1854

Puckett, J. A., Dyar, C., Maroney, M. R., Mustanski, B., & Newcomb, M. E. (2023). Daily experiences of minority stress and mental health in transgender and gender-diverse individuals. *Journal of Psychopathology and Clinical Science, 132*(3), 340–350. https://doi.org/10.1037/abn0000814

Puckett, J. A., Maroney, M. R., Mustanski, B., Newcomb, M. E., & Wadsworth, L. P. (2019). Coping with discrimination: The insidious effects of gender minority stigma on depression and anxiety in transgender individuals. *Journal of Clinical Psychology*, 1–19. https://doi.org/10.1002/jclp.22865

Puckett, J. A., Maroney, M. R., Wadsworth, L. P., Mustanski, B., & Newcomb, M. E. (2020). Coping with discrimination: The insidious effects of gender minority stigma on depression and anxiety in transgender individuals. *Journal of Clinical Psychology, 76*(1), 176–194. https://doi.org/10.1002/jclp.22865

Radusky, P. D., Zalazar, V., Cardozo, N., Fabian, S., Duarte, M., Frola, C., Cahn, P., Sued, O., & Aristegui, I. (2020). Reduction of gender identity stigma and improvements in mental health among transgender women initiating HIV treatment in a trans-sensitive clinic in Argentina. *Transgender Health, 5*(4), 216–224. https://doi.org/10.1089/trgh.2020.0005

Reisner, S. L., Poteat, T., Keatley, J., Cabral, M., Mothopeng, T., Dunham, E., & Baral, S. D. (2016). Global health burden and needs of transgender populations: A review. *The Lancet, 388*, 412–436. https://doi.org/10.1016/S0140-6736(16)00684-X

Restar, A. J., & Reisner, S. L. (2017). Protect trans people: Gender equality and equity in action. *The Lancet, 390*, 1933–1935. https://doi.org/10.1016/S0140-6736(17)31823-8

Ryan, C., Russell, S., Huebner, D., Diaz, R., & Sanchez, J. (2010). Family acceptance in adolescence and the health of LGBT young adults. *Journal of Child and Adolescent Psychiatric Nursing, 23*(4), 205–213. https://doi.org/10.1111/j.1744-6171.2010.00246.x

Sarno, E., Newcomb, M., & Mustanski, B. (2020). Rumination longitudinally mediates the association of minority stress and depression in sexual and gender minority individuals. *Journal of Abnormal Psychology, 129*(4), 355–363. https://doi.org/10.1037/abn0000508

Scandurra, C., Amodeo, A. L., Bochicchio, V., Valerio, P., & Frost, D. M. (2017a). Psychometric characteristics of the Transgender Identity Survey in an Italian sample: A measure to assess positive and negative feelings towards transgender identity. *International Journal of Transgenderism, 18*, 53–65. https://doi.org/10.1080/15532739.2016.1241975

Scandurra, C., Amodeo, A. L., Valerio, P., Bochicchio, V., & Frost, D. M. (2017b). Minority stress, resilience, and mental health: A study of Italian transgender people. *Journal of Social Issues, 73*, 563–585. https://doi.org/10.1111/josi.12232

Scandurra, C., Dolce, P., Vitelli, R., Esposito, G., Testa, R. J., Balsam, K. F., & Bochicchio, V. (2020). Mentalizing stigma: Reflective functioning as a protective factor against depression and anxiety in transgender and gender-nonconforming people. *Journal of Clinical Psychology, 76*, 1613–1630. https://doi.org/10.1002/jclp.22951

Scandurra, C., Vitelli, V., Maldonato, N. M., Valerio, P., & Bochicchio, V. (2019). A qualitative study on minority stress subjectively experienced by transgender and gender nonconforming people in Italy. *Sexologies: European Journal of Sexology and Sexual Health, 28*(3), e61–e71. https://doi.org/10.1016/j.sexol.2019.05.002

Scandurra, C., Bochicchio, V., Amodeo, A. L., Esposito, C., Valerio, P., Maldonato, N. M., Bacchini, D., & Vitelli, R. (2018). Internalized transphobia, resilience, and mental health: Applying the psychological mediation framework to Italian transgender individuals. *International Journal of Environmental Research and Public Health, 15*, 508. https://doi.org/10.3390/ijerph15030508

Sevelius, J. (2013). Gender affirmation: A framework for conceptualizing risk behavior among transgender women of color. *Sex Roles, 68*, 675–689. https://doi.org/10.1007/s11199-012-0216-5

Sevelius, J. M., Chakravarty, D., Dilworth, S. E., Rebchook, G., & Neilands, T. B. (2021). Measuring satisfaction and comfort with gender identity and gender expression among transgender women: Development and validation of the psychological gender affirmation scale. *International Journal of Environmental Research and Public Health, 18*(6), 1–13. https://doi.org/10.3390/ijerph18063298

Silva, G. W. D. S., Meira, K. C., Azevedo, D. M. D., Sena, R. C. F. D., Lins, S. L. D. F., Dantas, E. S. O., & Miranda, F. A. N. D. (2021). Fatores asso-ciados à ideação suicida entre travestis e transexuais assistidas por organizações não governamentais. *Cien. Saude Colet., 26*, 4955–4966. https://doi.org/10.3390/ijerph20043215

Snow, A., Cerel, J., Loeffler, D. N., & Flaherty, C. (2019). Barriers to mental health care for transgender and gender-nonconforming adults: A systematic literature review. *Health and Social Work, 44*(3), 149–155. https://doi.org/10.1093/hsw/hlz016

Soll, B. M., Robles-García, R., Brandelli-Costa, A., Mori, D., Mueller, A., Vaitses-Fontanari, A. M., Cardoso-da-Silva, D., Schwarz, K., Abel-Schneider, M., Saadeh, A., & Lobato, M. I. (2017). Gender incongruence: A comparative study using ICD-10 and DSM-5 diagnostic criteria. *Revista Brasileira de Psiquiatria, 40*(2), 174–180. https://doi.org/10.1590/1516-4446-2016-2224

Szymanski, D. M., Dunn, T. L., & Ikizler, A. S. (2014). Multiple minority stressors and psychological distress among sexual minority women: The roles of rumination and maladaptive coping. *Psychology of Sexual Orientation and Gender Diversity, 1*, 412–421. https://doi.org/10.1037/sgd0000066

Taliaferro, L. A., McMorris, B. J., & Eisenberg, M. E. (2018). Connections that moderate risk of non-suicidal self-injury among transgender and gender non-conforming youth. *Psychiatry Research, 268*, 65–67. https://doi.org/10.1016/j.psychres.2018.06.068

Tan, K., Treharne, G., Ellis, S., Schmidt, J., & Veale, J. (2020). Gender minority stress: A critical review. *Journal of Homosexuality, 67*(10), 1471–1489. https://doi.org/10.1080/00918369.2019.1591789

Testa, R. J., Habarth, J., Peta, J., Balsam, J., & Bockting, W. O. (2015). Development of the gender minority stress and resilience measure. *Psychology of Sexual Orientation and Gender Diversity, 2*, 65–77. https://doi.org/10.1037/sgd0000081

The Trevor Project. (2023). *2023 U.S. national survey on the mental health of LGBTQ young people.* : The Trevor Project. https://www.thetrevorproject.org/survey-2023/

Tomicic, A., Martínez, C., Rodríguez, J., & Barrientos, J. (2024). *Informe Final Proyecto Fondecyt: Desarrollo de un Modelo Comprensivo de Psicoterapia con Pacientes LGBT: Estudio Cualitativo de las Experiencias de Pacientes y de Psicoterapeutas [Final Project Report: Development of a Comprehensive Psychotherapy Model with LGBT Patients: Qualitative Study of the Experiences of Patients and Psychotherapists].* Proyecto Fondecyt Regular N°1190270. ANID.

Tucker, R. P. (2019). Suicide in transgender veterans: Prevalence, prevention, and implications of current policy. *Perspectives on Psychological Science, 14*(3), 452–468. https://doi.org/10.1177/1745691618812680

Virupaksha, H. G., Muralidhar, D., & Ramakrishna, J. (2016). Suicide and suicidal behavior among transgender persons. *Indian Journal of Psychological Medicine, 38*, 505–509. https://doi.org/10.4103/0253-7176.194908

Wilson, L. C., & Liss, M. (2022). Belonging and loneliness as mechanisms in the psychological impact of discrimination among transgender college students. *Journal of LGBT Youth*. Advance online publication. https://doi.org/10.1080/19361653.2022.2049418

Zwickl, S., Wong, A., Dowers, E., Leemaqz, Y., Bretherton, I., Cook, T., Zajac, J., Yip, P., & Cheung, A. (2021). Factors associated with suicide attempts among Australian transgender adults – external site opens in a new window. *BMC Psychiatry, 21*, 81. https://doi.org/10.1186/s12888-021-03084-7

Chapter 6
Understanding Suicidal Behavior in the Context of Mapuche Culture

Reiner Fuentes-Ferrada, Margarita Morandé, and Tomás Baader

6.1 Cultural Considerations in the Study of Indigenous Suicide

International research shows that Indigenous youth exhibit higher rates of suicidal behavior compared to their non-Indigenous peers. This pattern has been observed across various groups, including Sami youth in Sweden (Omma et al., 2013; Eckhoff et al., 2020), American Indian and Alaska Native adolescents (Qiao & Bell, 2017), Canadian Indigenous youth (Webster, 2016), and the Maori population in New Zealand (Beautrais & Fergusson, 2006).

The study of Indigenous suicidal behavior requires new frameworks of understanding within Western suicidology (Ansloos, 2018). Recent research suggests that there should be a focus on cultural knowledge and Indigenous spirituality (Rowe & Ansloos, 2024; Richardson & Waters, 2023), as well as the impact of historical trauma and colonization processes (Brockie et al., 2024; Ehlers et al., 2022; Barnhart & May, 2021). Recognizing the epistemological and methodological differences between healthcare teams and Indigenous communities is crucial (de Almeida et al., 2024; Kovach, 2010).

R. Fuentes-Ferrada (✉)
Faculty of Psychology, University of Valencia, Valencia, Spain

Alianza Chilena Contra la Depresión, Valdivia, Chile

Nucleus to Improve the Mental Health of Adolescents and Youths (Imhay), Santiago, Chile
e-mail: reifuen@alumni.uv.es

M. Morandé
Faculty of Psychology and Humanities, Universidad San Sebastián, Valdivia, Chile

Alianza Chilena Contra la Depresión, Valdivia, Chile

T. Baader
Alianza Chilena Contra la Depresión, Valdivia, Chile

Á. Jiménez-Molina, V. Martínez (eds.), *New Perspectives on Suicidal Behavior, Depression and Personality*, https://doi.org/10.1007/978-3-031-96037-6_6

Suicide prevention programs in Indigenous contexts have often neglected cultural variables, focusing instead on individual factors rather than family or community aspects (Sjoblom et al., 2022). Interventions must align with Indigenous health paradigms, emphasizing a strong community and family component (Barker et al., 2017). A culturally respectful approach to suicide involves understanding the cultural representations and meanings associated with it from the Indigenous worldview.

Suicide mortality among the Mapuche people, one of the nine officially recognized Indigenous groups, is higher than in the non-Mapuche population, particularly among young people. For instance, in southern Chile, 40% of suicides among the Mapuche occur in individuals under 30 years old, compared to 20% in the non-Mapuche population (Oyarce & Pedrero, 2011). This disparity is also reflected in suicide attempts. According to the Unit for People with Suicidal Attempts (UPI) at the Valdivia Base Hospital, 12.9% of those who made one or more suicide attempts in the Los Ríos Region identified as belonging to the Mapuche people (Gotelli et al., 2023).

In Mapuche culture, health is understood as *Küme Mogñen* or "Buen Vivir" (Good Living), a concept representing holistic well-being based on the balance between the individual, the community, and the ecosystem (Torres et al., 1995). This balance is achieved through the *Ad-Mapu*, a set of ancestral norms and values that govern Mapuche's behavior, encompassing moral, spiritual, and social aspects. Illness, in this context, can stem from natural, supernatural, or social causes, such as discrimination, cultural disconnection, or the violation of traditions (*Kutran*). To illustrate Mapuche's understanding of suicide, this chapter presents two experiences: a community encounter with Mapuche communities in southern Chile and a therapeutic encounter with a Mapuche clinical case at risk of suicide.

6.2 A Community Gathering with Mapuche Culture on Suicide

In 2018, two discussions, known as "*trawun*" in *Mapudungun*, were held to deepen the understanding of suicide from the Mapuche perspective and gather their insights. These meetings, conducted in the Los Ríos region of Chile, focused on exchanging knowledge about health and illness processes, as well as the Mapuche view on suicide. Key questions were discussed using a focus group methodology, such as: How does Mapuche culture understand health? What factors cause illness? How do Mapuche communities perceive suicide?

These discussions were attended by important Mapuche figures, including *Machis*, who play a crucial role in Mapuche culture by managing medical-religious knowledge and acting as intermediaries with the spiritual world, and *lawentuchefes*, recognized in the community for their healing role based on knowledge of herbal medicine. Cultural facilitators and Indigenous leaders from various Mapuche communities in the region also participated.

Among the main findings, it is noted that Mapuche culture perceives health as an inseparable connection between the psychic, physical, and territorial dimensions while also incorporating spiritual and environmental aspects. This holistic approach ties well-being to a balance in the relationship with nature, culture, and the spiritual world, where disruption can negatively impact health.

Regarding suicide, four explanatory perspectives were identified that reflect the comprehensive understanding of well-being in Mapuche communities:

- Spiritual perspective: A malevolent spirit takes control of the body.
- Cultural perspective: Suicide results from the transgression of a cultural norm.
- Family perspective: There is a generational predisposition, where if an ancestor died by suicide, another family member might do the same.
- Health perspective: Changes in mood and behavior related to depressive symptoms.

These perspectives are not mutually exclusive and can intersect to make sense of the loss of a community member to suicide.

From the health perspective, specific risk indicators for Mapuche men were identified due to their tendency to express emotions less openly, making it more challenging to detect suicide risk. These indicators include social isolation, alcohol consumption, changes in oral expressiveness toward more silent behavior, and difficulties in fulfilling expected cultural roles, such as working the land, participating in religious ceremonies, and passing on knowledge orally. These factors align with some described in Western literature, particularly the link between suicide and problematic substance use, which has been highlighted as one of the most significant harms to Indigenous communities in the Americas (PAHO, 2016).

While it is possible to identify common risk factors between Indigenous and non-Indigenous populations, these are often viewed from an individual, biological, or psychological perspective. However, in Indigenous communities, it is essential to recognize that these factors stem from unique historical and cultural contexts. Social and cultural phenomena that generate intersubjective distress, such as historical trauma—encompassing community and individual pain passed down through generations due to environmental damage, symbolic violence, and racism—are present across different Indigenous communities (Walters, 2006).

6.3 An Encounter with the Mapuche Spiritual World

This section details a nearly decade-long therapeutic process in which the significance of Mapuche and Western Christian worldviews, inherited from the patient's family, gradually came to light. Javiera, an elementary school teacher, first sought psychiatric help at the age of 36 in 2009. Despite her generally cheerful demeanor, she experienced significant internal distress. She was diagnosed with panic disorder and anxiety and was prescribed anxiolytics alongside cognitive-behavioral therapy. Initially, Javiera attributed her symptoms—such as tachycardia, chest tightness, and fear of dying—to "grief" and work-related stress. These episodes, lasting between 30 min and an hour, exhausted her.

In the early months of treatment, the focus was on managing her panic attacks. Javiera recognized certain aspects of her personality, such as her desire for acceptance, particularly from her parents. Her mother, from a conservative Catholic English family, was highly demanding, while her father, of Mapuche origin, was a respected local historian deeply connected to literature and poetry. Over time, Javiera began to experience episodes of distress and mood fluctuations unrelated to her panic attacks. These cycles included periods of depression, anhedonia, and difficulty concentrating, followed by phases of heightened self-esteem, increased activity, reduced sleep, and a surge of energy. Further investigation revealed a history of mood disorders on her father's side, leading to a diagnosis of bipolar II disorder and the initiation of mood-stabilizing treatment.

Three years into her treatment, Javiera began to explore deeper aspects of her life, including her belief in witchcraft. She revealed that she had been visiting a *Machi*, a spiritual leader in her community, who explained that her distress stemmed from not following her ancestral calling to become a *Machi*. Javiera shared that she had been having spiritual dreams, known as *Peuma*, since childhood, in which her ancestors revealed that she was destined to continue the family tradition of being a *Machi*.

As Javiera delved deeper into her cultural heritage, she visited a Mapuche community in southern Chile, where she was received by the *Lonco* (community leader), who had been expecting her. This visit intensified her dreams and strengthened her connection to the ancestral world. During this period, Javiera remained stable in her bipolar treatment, and the therapy respected and incorporated her cultural worldview, acknowledging the significance of her *Peumas* and her calling to become a *Machi*. During this time, Javiera's maternal family noticed changes in her, such as distraction and strange dreams, prompting them to take her to a health center. She was referred to Psychiatry with a possible diagnosis of schizophrenia. However, an Ecuadorian psychiatrist in training understood the cultural context of her experiences and dismissed this diagnosis.

Javiera continued her treatment with the *Machi*, who guided her through a spiritual healing process. The *Machi* advised her to distance herself from her family of origin and establish herself in the Indigenous community to assume her role as a *Machi*. Although this advice caused tension for Javiera, she reconnected with her roots and developed a project to support Mapuche communities.

In 2013, Javiera achieved a state of euthymia through pharmacological and therapeutic treatment. During this period, she interrupted her relationship with the *Machi* and stopped taking the medicinal herbs recommended for her healing. This interruption led her to confront childhood traumas, including a forced abortion at the age of 16 by a manipulative ex-partner, which profoundly affected her emotional life and relationships.

At the end of 2014, Javiera experienced a deep existential void, accompanied by tachycardia and anxiety, although less intense than her previous panic attacks. In early 2015, she sought spiritual guidance from a monk of the Benedictine Order, beginning a healing process. During this time, Javiera achieved a synthesis between her Mapuche and Christian beliefs. Through prayer and exorcism rituals, she overcame intense experiences of dreams with demonic figures, feeling more stable and at peace afterward. However, the diagnosis of her father's dementia and the suicide of a young Mapuche man she knew deeply affected her. Javiera resumed antidepressant treatment for a short period. Reflecting on suicide within Mapuche culture, she noted that this act disrupts the transmission of ancestral knowledge, harming not only the community but also the family's descendants and breaking the ancestral bond that maintains the community's social and spiritual balance.

At the beginning of 2016, Javiera mentioned that she remained in contact with the monk, who even visited her in the city where she lived, continuing the spiritual healing process in the Christian aspect of her life. This connection led her to embark on a trip to a Third World Poor Foundation run by an Augustinian nuns' congregation. She spent a few months in an orphanage in Cusco, Peru, in March and May 2016. The experience was intense for her, as the extreme poverty and lack of basic hygienic living conditions in the neighborhood where she volunteered deeply impacted her. She was struck by the nuns' vocation, mysticism, and spirituality integrated into their work, making the experience profoundly enriching both relationally and spiritually for Javiera. Upon returning to southern Chile, she entered a period of mood instability, reconnecting with traumatic memories of the forced abortion at 16, which she still recalls with guilt. This was one of the most challenging phases, marked by increased mood instability, frequent suicidal ideation, and a well-formed plan to end her life, leading to an emergency hospitalization. Overwhelmed by the suffering in her life, she felt that it might be better not to exist.

In subsequent outpatient visits, Javiera stabilized and seriously considered following her ancestral Mapuche vocation, dedicating herself to healing others. This purpose allowed her to reconnect with her *Peumas*, where her ancestors urged her to become a "healer," providing her peace and direction.

In October 2016, she was involved in a car accident, resulting in a mild to moderate traumatic brain injury with a brief loss of consciousness. After fully recovering in the following weeks, Javiera experienced a profound change, reconnecting with the value of life and strengthening her resolve to help others. Following this event, she began working at an intercultural center in a nature reserve near Lake Panguipulli, where she assumed the role of *Ñampin*, a Mapuche figure who assesses individuals' emotional and spiritual state and offers treatments for their recovery. From that time until early 2021, she did not attend regular check-ups. Table 6.1 summarizes the spiritual and therapeutic support received and the significant events.

This therapeutic encounter reveals how, from the Mapuche worldview, there is an etiological explanation of suicide linked to lineage and the vocation of becoming a *Machi*. The process of becoming a *Machi* often involves behaviors and manifestations that can be mistaken for psychotic symptoms. However, these are not permanent and do not hinder social integration within the cultural context. Being a *Machi* requires sacrificing personal projects for the community's well-being, which is challenging. In treating this case, it was crucial to validate Mapuche cultural practices, such as dreams or *Peumas*, interpreted by the *Machi*, who serve as a bridge

Table 6.1 Spiritual and therapeutic support and significant events and experiences

Age	Support	Events, experiences
10–12 years old 16 years old	No support	Sexual abuse Forced abortion and intimate partner violence
36 years old	Start of therapeutic process	Divorce, work-related stress, and onset of panic attacks
40 years old	Discontinuation of *Machi's* support	Onset of traumatic memories
42 years old	Beginning of Christian spiritual support	Suicide of a young Mapuche person Acute suicidality and hospitalization
43 years old	Christian volunteer trip	Car accident Begins role as *Ñampin*
48 years old	Discontinuation of therapeutic process	

between the natural and spiritual worlds. Connecting with the land and culture strengthened the patient's identity, leading to improvement as she integrated her two worlds—the Mapuche and the Christian Catholic. This syncretism, supported by the *Machi* and a monk, reinforced her gift and deepened her connection with family traditions.

Javiera's case emphasizes the importance of a comprehensive approach in therapeutic care, avoiding premature diagnoses. It is crucial to respect each person's cultural experiences and meanings and consider their cultural context during evaluation. This ethical stance is essential for healthcare teams promoting well-being within Indigenous communities.

6.4 Toward an Intercultural Suicidology

Understanding suicide requires considering both the social structure and the cultural frameworks that shape the experience. It is essential to analyze how experiential, psychological, social, and cultural factors interact within local contexts (Kirmayer, 2022). Qualitative research can contribute to this understanding by revealing how cultural meanings, institutions, and practices support interpersonal interactions and influence broader structural processes that shape personal experience and a sense of agency (Hjelmeland, 2012).

From the Mapuche worldview, suicide is seen as a multifactorial phenomenon that encompasses the relationship with nature, spiritual beings, and the acceptance or rejection of roles within the community. In Javiera's case, three key cultural aspects that may influence Indigenous suicidality were identified. First, the tension between accepting a spiritual role imposed by lineage and the community, such as becoming a *Machi*, and maintaining Western roles, such as being a mother and teacher, can create constant psychological distress. The discrepancies between

Western lifestyles and spiritual roles within the community may increase the risk of suicidality (Azuero et al., 2017). Second, spiritual struggles, whether in the form of faith crises or conflicts with spiritual beings (Pargament & Exline, 2023), are experiences that can be linked to suicidal ideation and suicide risk (Lemke et al., 2023; Currier et al., 2018). Third, suicide planning can be triggered after exposure to the suicide of a young Mapuche, as suicide contagion in Indigenous communities presents unique characteristics compared to Western contexts (Derek Cheung et al., 2014; Hanssens, 2016).

To effectively address suicidality in Indigenous contexts, it is essential to integrate community-based healing practices with Western treatments. This requires, first and foremost, epistemological humility from professionals to embrace experiences that fall outside traditional frameworks, such as the calling to be a *Machi* or mystical experiences, which could be misinterpreted as psychotic symptoms. Second, it is important to consider family, community, and social variables beyond individual factors, as sociohistorical processes like industrialization or environmental degradation can contribute to a "cultural death" associated with suicide in Indigenous populations (Azuero et al., 2017). Third, validating the spiritual and religious knowledge of the community in treatment is crucial. Additionally, it is necessary to recognize the distinction in Mapuche culture between illnesses of Mapuche origin and those of Western origin, which should be considered when defining treatment procedures in both medical systems.

Finally, it is essential to move beyond the limitations of Western suicidology, which often views suicide as an individual pathology focused on psychological risk factors (White, 2017). To effectively address suicidal behaviors from an intercultural perspective, it is crucial to adopt a contextual approach that incorporates cultural competencies and promotes dialogue between different cultures. This integrative approach will enhance therapeutic resources and provide a deeper understanding of human suffering across diverse cultural contexts.

Acknowledgment RF-F received funding from ANID—Millennium Science Initiative Program—NCS2021_081—International Doctoral Scholarship 2024 - 72240072.

References

Ansloos, J. (2018). Rethinking Indigenous suicide. *International Journal of Indigenous Health, 13*(2), 8–28. https://doi.org/10.32799/ijih.v13i2.32061

Azuero, A. J., Arreaza-Kaufman, D., Coriat, J., Tassinari, S., Faria, A., Castañeda-Cardona, C., & Rosselli, D. (2017). Suicide in the indigenous population of Latin America: A systematic review. *Revista Colombiana de Psiquiatria, 46*(4), 237–242. https://doi.org/10.1016/j.rcp.2016.12.002

Barker, B., Goodman, A., & DeBeck, K. (2017). Reclaiming Indigenous identities: Culture as strength against suicide among Indigenous youth in Canada. *Canadian Journal of Public Health = Revue canadienne de sante publique, 108*(2), e208–e210. https://doi.org/10.17269/cjph.108.5754

Barnhart, G., & May, A. D. (2021). A historical and contextual review of the adverse psychological effects of the trauma of colonialization on Alaska native peoples. *Psychology from the Margins, 3*(1), 2.

Beautrais, A. L., & Fergusson, D. M. (2006). Indigenous suicide in New Zealand. *Archives of Suicide Research: Official Journal of the International Academy for Suicide Research, 10*(2), 159–168. https://doi.org/10.1080/13811110600556913

Brockie, T., Kahn-John, M., Mata Lopez, L., Decker, E., Glass, N., Kazemi, M., Perez-Monteau, R., Miryck, A., Nelson, K., Ricker, A., Rider, T., Roberts, T., Wilson, D., Yazzie, K., & Perrin, N. (2024). A mixed-methods study protocol on factors contributing to suicide clusters among Native American youth in a northern plains reservation. *Frontiers in Public Health, 11*, 1281109. https://doi.org/10.3389/fpubh.2023.1281109

Currier, J. M., McDermott, R. C., McCormick, W. H., Churchwell, M. C., & Milkeris, L. (2018). Exploring cross-lagged associations between spiritual struggles and risk for suicidal behavior in a community sample of military veterans. *Journal of Affective Disorders, 230*, 93–100. https://doi.org/10.1016/j.jad.2018.01.009

de Almeida, M. N., Caixeta, C. C., Santos Silva, N. D., de Morais, N. M., Dos Santos, P. D., Gonçalves, L. P., Achatz, R. W., Silva Guimarães, D., & Chaudhary, N. (2024). Challenges and concerns in assisting indigenous people with suicide attempts. *Integrative Psychological & Behavioral Science, 58*(1), 319–337. https://doi.org/10.1007/s12124-023-09803-x

Derek Cheung, Y. T., Spittal, M. J., Williamson, M. K., Tung, S. J., & Pirkis, J. (2014). Predictors of suicides occurring within suicide clusters in Australia, 2004-2008. *Social Science & Medicine (1982), 118*, 135–142. https://doi.org/10.1016/j.socscimed.2014.08.005

Eckhoff, C., Sørvold, M. T., & Kvernmo, S. (2020). Adolescent self-harm and suicidal behavior and young adult outcomes in Indigenous and non-Indigenous people. *European Child & Adolescent Psychiatry, 29*(7), 917–927. https://doi.org/10.1007/s00787-019-01406-5

Ehlers, C. L., Yehuda, R., Gilder, D. A., Bernert, R., & Karriker-Jaffe, K. J. (2022). Trauma, historical trauma, PTSD and suicide in an American Indian community sample. *Journal of Psychiatric Research, 156*, 214–220. https://doi.org/10.1016/j.jpsychires.2022.10.012

Gotelli, M., Manríquez, J., Zambrano, C., Yañez, E., & Fuentes-Ferrada, R. (2023). Clinical and sociodemographic characterization of the suicide attempt in the Los Ríos Region, Chile. *Revista chilena de neuro-psiquiatría, 61*(1), 32–42. https://doi.org/10.4067/S0717-92272023000100032

Hanssens, L. (2016). The impact of suicide contagion and intergenerational segregation on youth and young adults in remote Indigenous communities in Northern Territory, Australia. *Aboriginal and Islander Health Worker Journal, 40*, 38–47.

Hjelmeland, H. (2012). Suicide research and prevention: The importance of culture in "biological times". In E. Colucci, D. Lester, H. Hjelmeland, & B. C. B. Park (Eds.), *Suicide and culture: Understanding the context* (pp. 3–18). Hogrefe.

Kirmayer, L. J. (2022). Suicide in cultural context: An ecosocial approach. *Transcultural Psychiatry, 59*(1), 3–12. https://doi.org/10.1177/13634615221076424

Kovach, M. (2010). *Indigenous methodologies: Characteristics, conversations, and contexts*. University of Toronto Press.

Lemke, A. W., Davis, E. B., Voytenko, V. L., Cowden, R. G., Chen, Z. J., McConnell, J. M., Pargament, K., Phillips, K., Marseilles, R., & Wolff, R. P. (2023). Religious/spiritual struggles and suicide ideation among adult psychiatric outpatients: A 12-month longitudinal study. *Journal of Affective Disorders Reports, 14*, 100640. https://doi.org/10.1016/j.jadr.2023.100640

Omma, L., Sandlund, M., & Jacobsson, L. (2013). Suicidal expressions in young Swedish Sami, a cross-sectional study. *International Journal of Circumpolar Health, 72*. https://doi.org/10.3402/ijch.v72i0.19862

Organización Paramericana de Salud. (2016). *Promoción de la Salud Mental en Población Indigenas. Experiencias de Países*. Oficina Regional para las Américas de la Organización Mundial de la Salud.

Oyarce, A., & Pedrero, M. (2011). *Perfil epidemiológico de la población mapuche residente en el área de cobertura del Servicio de Salud Provincia del Bío-Bío*. Serie análisis de estudios de salud de los pueblos indígenas de Chile. Región del Bío-Bío N° 1. Ministerio de Salud.

Pargament, K. I., & Exline, J. J. (2023). Shaken to the core: Understanding and addressing spiritual struggles in psychotherapy. In P. S. Richards, G. E. K. Allen, & D. K. Judd (Eds.), *Handbook of spiritually integrated psychotherapies* (pp. 119–133). American Psychological Association. https://doi.org/10.1037/0000338-006

Qiao, N., & Bell, T. M. (2017). Indigenous adolescents' suicidal behaviors and risk factors: Evidence from the National Youth Risk Behavior Survey. *Journal of Immigrant and Minority Health, 19*(3), 590–597. https://doi.org/10.1007/s10903-016-0443-x

Richardson, M., & Waters, S. F. (2023). Indigenous voices against suicide: A meta-synthesis advancing prevention strategies. *International Journal of Environmental Research and Public Health, 20*(22), 7064. https://doi.org/10.3390/ijerph20227064

Rowe, S., & Ansloos, J. P. (2024). Understanding suicide from an indigenous cultural lens: Insights from elders in Canada. *Journal of Religion and Health, 63*(2), 1038–1057. https://doi.org/10.1007/s10943-024-02022-7

Sjoblom, E., Ghidei, W., Leslie, M., James, A., Bartel, R., Campbell, S., & Montesanti, S. (2022). Centering Indigenous knowledge in suicide prevention: A critical scoping review. *BMC Public Health, 22*(1), 2377. https://doi.org/10.1186/s12889-022-14580-0

Torres, C., Conejeros, A. M., & Jelves, I. (1995). *Manual de salud para áreas rurales mapuches*. Imprenta Austral.

Walters, K. (2006). Indigenous perspectives in survey research: Conceptualising and measuring historical trauma, microaggressions, and colonial trauma response. *Mātauranga taketake: Traditional knowledge. Indigenous indicators of well-being: Perspectives, practices, solutions* (pp. 27–44).

Webster, P. C. (2016). Canada's Indigenous suicide crisis. *Lancet (London, England), 387*(10037), 2494. https://doi.org/10.1016/S0140-6736(16)30836-4

White, J. (2017). What can critical suicidology do? *Death Studies, 41*(8), 472–480. https://doi.org/10.1080/07481187.2017.1332901

Part II
Clinical Assessment and Psychosocial Interventions

Chapter 7
Comprehensive Understanding of Young People Suicide Risk Assessment and Intervention

Vania Martínez and Belén Vargas

7.1 Young People Suicide Risk

According to the World Health Organization (WHO, 2024), suicide is the third most common cause of death among individuals aged 15–29. Beyond the statistics, each suicide represents a tragedy that profoundly impacts families, communities, and society. Moreover, for every suicide death, many more young people attempt suicide, and even more experience suicidal ideation (World Health Organization, 2024). Both suicide attempts and suicidal ideation are significant risk factors for suicide death and are associated with long-term adverse outcomes (Cantor et al., 2023).

While the long-term impact of the COVID-19 pandemic on suicide risk among young people is still not fully understood, preliminary data indicate a general increase in these cases (Goto et al., 2022; Kim et al., 2024; Maciá-Casas et al., 2024). Experiences of grief, disruptions in routine and social interactions, and an

V. Martínez (✉)
Faculty of Medicine, Universidad de Chile, Santiago, RM - Santiago, Chile

Nucleus to Improve the Mental Health of Adolescents and Youths (Imhay), Santiago, Chile

Mental Health Department, Ministerio de Salud, Santiago, Chile

Millennium Institute for Research in Depression and Personality (MIDAP), Santiago, Chile
e-mail: vmartinezn@uchile.cl

B. Vargas
Nucleus to Improve the Mental Health of Adolescents and Youths (Imhay), Santiago, Chile

Mental Health Department, Ministerio de Salud, Santiago, Chile

Doctoral Program in Psychotherapy, Universidad de Chile and Pontificia Universidad Católica de Chile, Santiago, Chile

Á. Jiménez-Molina, V. Martínez (eds.), *New Perspectives on Suicidal Behavior*, Depression and Personality, https://doi.org/10.1007/978-3-031-96037-6_7

increase in depression and anxiety symptoms could raise the suicide risk in this population (Goto et al., 2022).

These findings highlight the need for implementing prevention strategies, early detection initiatives, and timely management of suicide risk cases among young people. However, significant barriers hinder access to mental health professionals for young people at risk of suicide, creating a considerable treatment gap (Bruffaerts et al., 2019). Even when young people at risk of suicide gain access to treatment, their management can be very challenging. A clear and thorough approach to risk assessment and developing an appropriate treatment plan is required.

This chapter is organized into four sections. The first explores key risk and protective factors for youth suicide, emphasizing the importance of considering social determinants of health and providing a broad perspective on the complexities of suicide risk and resilience in young populations. The second section focuses on tools for screening and assessing suicide risk, offering an overview of recommended instruments and practical approaches. The following section highlights interventions applicable in clinical, community, and digital settings. Strategies include primary healthcare-based approaches, educational environments, and digital solutions like apps and online platforms designed to extend accessibility and scalability of support. Finally, the chapter examines the structural and attitudinal barriers hindering young people's help-seeking behaviors.

By offering a panorama view of these key areas, the chapter aims to contribute to developing more accessible, effective, and sustainable comprehension and prevention of suicide risk for young populations.

7.2 Risk and Protective Factors

Identifying risk factors for young people is a contribution since it facilitates the orientation of interventions aimed at those with greater vulnerability, making it possible to address preventable or modifiable aspects. At the same time, recognizing protective factors contributes to a more comprehensive assessment and favors implementing preventive interventions.

Risk and protective factors for suicide in young people share many similarities with those in adults. However, the particularities of youth development may intensify the impact of certain factors, such as decision-making, coping strategies, family and peer relationships, and victimization (Wasserman et al., 2021).

The relatively infrequent nature of suicide and its complex etiology make it challenging to identify predictors of suicide attempts and suicide with reasonable levels of sensitivity and specificity. For example, although there is a high correlation between suicide and a psychiatric diagnosis, most people with a psychiatric diagnosis do not die by suicide or attempt suicide (Melvin et al., 2023). Thus, the goal is not to predict suicide with certainty but rather to identify and support those at most significant risk through comprehensive prevention strategies and early intervention.

7.2.1 Risk Factors

Risk factors for suicidal behavior can be described as correlates that precede both suicide and suicide ideation and attempt (Franklin et al., 2017). Suicide risk is multifactorial and involves factors at the individual, family, peer, and community levels. Consequently, these factors can be categorized and identified as follows (Hawton et al., 2022; Ruch et al., 2024):

- Individual level: Mental health problems, substance abuse, previous suicidal behaviors, history of trauma, physical and sexual abuse, medical illnesses, impulsivity or aggression, and belonging to sexual orientation and gender identity minorities
- Family level: Conflicting family, family violence, family loss, family stress, family history of mental health disorders, and family history of suicide
- Peer level: Conflicting peer relationships, interpersonal loss, bullying, and cyberbullying
- Community level: Lack of supportive relationships, barriers to accessing healthcare services, access to lethal means, and unsafe portrayals of suicide in the media

Another way to classify risk factors is according to their temporality and proximity to suicidal behavior (Misiak et al., 2023). Distal risk factors are those background and long-term factors that elevate the chronic risk of suicide. In contrast, proximal factors are current and acute, increase risk in the present, and can be triggers for suicidal behavior.

Among the distal factors with the most scientific evidence is sex, where males have a higher risk of dying by suicide beginning at puberty. In comparison, females have a higher risk of suicidal ideation and suicide attempts. However, increasing concern has been noted about rising suicide rates among adolescent females (Ruch et al., 2019). Age is another key distal factor, with suicide rates increasing progressively from early adolescence to adulthood. Belonging to minoritized population groups, such as the Indigenous population, migrants, racialized groups, and LGBT+ persons, also elevates risk. Additional distal factors include a history of early adverse events (e.g., sexual and physical abuse) and personal experiences of suicidal ideation, suicide attempts, and self-inflicted injuries without suicidal intent (Hawton et al., 2022; Hughes et al., 2023; Melvin et al., 2023; Misiak et al., 2023; Wasserman et al., 2021).

Furthermore, psychiatric diagnoses such as mood disorders, schizophrenia, anxiety disorders, posttraumatic stress disorder, alcohol and substance use disorders, borderline personality disorder, and neurodevelopmental disorders, among others, contribute to the risk. This risk increases significantly in cases of comorbidity, where two or more mental health disorders coexist. A family history of mental health disorders or suicide represents another important distal risk factor (Hawton et al., 2022; Hughes et al., 2023; Melvin et al., 2023; Misiak et al., 2023; Wasserman et al., 2021).

The most frequently mentioned proximal factors in the literature include psychiatric and psychological symptoms such as aggression, impulsivity, psychotic-like experiences, insomnia, intense anxiety or agitation, feelings of entrapment, purposelessness, hopelessness, and depressed mood. Other significant risk factors include the period following discharge from psychiatric hospitalization or an emergency department visit for suicidal or self-injurious behavior, problematic use of alcohol and other substances, and medical diagnoses—especially when associated with physical pain or stigma (Hawton et al., 2022; Hughes et al., 2023; Melvin et al., 2023; Misiak et al., 2023; Wasserman et al., 2021).

Additionally, experiences of bullying, victimization, or trauma, as well as interpersonal conflicts, financial or personal losses, and adverse life circumstances linked to shame, humiliation, or rejection, further increase the risk. Access to suicide methods, the suicide of a close or admired person, significant anniversaries, social isolation, and lack of a support network are also identified as key proximal factors (Hawton et al., 2022; Hughes et al., 2023; Melvin et al., 2023; Misiak et al., 2023; Wasserman et al., 2021).

In addressing suicidal risk, it is important to consider that there are risk factors that are potentially modifiable (such as lack of support network and access to lethal means) or preventable (such as bullying). Furthermore, from the theory of intersectionality, it is postulated that social categories such as sex, race or ethnicity, socioeconomic status, gender identity, and sexual orientation intersect, reflecting multiple individual attributes and social contexts that influence health and risk behaviors (Bauer et al., 2021). Thus, awareness of intersectional inequalities provides a framework for understanding the various social factors that may contribute to suicide risk in youth (Hughes et al., 2023).

7.2.2 Protective Factors

Identifying and prioritizing protective factors for suicide is essential for timely intervention (Bakken et al., 2024; Hawton et al., 2022; Hughes et al., 2023; Melvin et al., 2023; Wasserman et al., 2021). The suicide protective factors identified in the literature can be categorized as follows:

- Motivations for living: Affective bonds (family, friends, loved ones, pets); goals and aspirations (having dreams and future goals, hope for upcoming events)
- Deterrents: Concern about the consequences; fear of death or severe injury; cultural, spiritual, and religious beliefs that discourage suicide and reinforce self-preservation
- Psychological and emotional well-being: Life satisfaction and positive self-image (self-esteem, perceived social competence, and satisfaction with physical appearance); effective clinical mental health care and positive therapeutic relationships

- Adaptive coping strategies: Reduced reliance on emotion-focused coping strategies; emotional regulation; cognitive flexibility; problem-solving skills; conflict resolution; adaptability to change; tolerance for ambiguity, stress, and frustration; help-seeking
- Support networks and connectedness: Family support networks (cohesion and emotional support); social support and access to services (interaction with the community and helping resources); connectedness to the environment (sense of belonging to family, school or college, community, and culture)

7.2.3 Social Determinants

From a public health perspective, broader contextual factors that influence individuals' health levels can be identified and shaped by political, social, and economic forces. These factors, known as social determinants of health, refer to the circumstances in which people's lives unfold, shaped by structural mechanisms of unequal power distribution and social stratification (World Health Organization Commission on Social Determinants of Health, 2008). Social determinants of health create and perpetuate health inequities, limiting opportunities for young people and groups to enjoy their right to health and access necessary care in the face of illness (Lund et al., 2018; Marmot et al., 2008; Salinas-Contreras et al., 2023).

Social determinants of health have a direct or indirect impact on the significant risk factors for suicide at the individual level, including sociodemographic factors (e.g., age, sex, education, employment, and income), contextual factors (e.g., stressful life events, suicide bereavement, and access to methods used for suicide), and clinical factors (such as mental illness, drug and alcohol use, history of suicide attempts, and chronic physical illness), as well as personality-related, genetic or familial, and neurobiological factors (Pirkis et al., 2024b).

Among the social determinants of health associated with suicidal behavior and ideation, several factors during adolescence and youth have been identified, including encounters with the justice system, experiences in foster care, exposure to maltreatment and abuse (such as child and sexual abuse), and belonging to sexual orientation and gender identity minorities (Na et al., 2025).

Identifying key social determinants that increase suicide risk in specific groups enables their prioritization in public policy and large-scale preventive strategies

7.3 Screening and Assessment

Early detection of suicide risk in young people is a fundamental step in its prevention, although many cases go unnoticed. Establishing a therapeutic relationship is the first task for professionals treating patients with suicidal ideation, even before assessing risk. This can be challenging due to patient ambivalence, previous negative experiences, severity of illness, and the need for immediate clinical assessment. Proper techniques include empathic listening, validation of feelings, and a collaborative approach (Melvin et al., 2023)

Many young people who die by suicide visit health services weeks or months beforehand. Primary healthcare providers can initiate important conversations with brief, evidence-based tools (Ruch et al., 2024). There is concern that asking young people about suicide may "put ideas in their heads." However, several studies have refuted this myth, demonstrating that asking these questions does not cause harm (Mathias et al., 2012).

It is critical to distinguish between "screening," which quickly identifies those who need further evaluation, and "assessment," which confirms risk and guides the next steps. Both are essential to an effective suicide prevention strategy (Hughes et al., 2023).

There is debate about the value of universal screening (population-wide) versus selective screening (in higher-risk subgroups). Selective screening allows for more efficient use of resources by focusing on individuals at higher risk, potentially leading to earlier detection and intervention in those most likely to benefit. However, universal screening can improve equity by eliminating bias and reducing healthcare access barriers (Hughes et al., 2023). In any case, it is recommended to start the screenings at age 12 years as part of regular preventive checkups and in children younger than 12 years when there are clinical clues, such as mental health problems or a history of suicidal thoughts and behaviors (American Academy of Pediatrics, 2022).

Suicide is closely related to depression, and screening for depression is often the first step in suicide prevention in primary healthcare settings. One instrument that stands out for its good performance in terms of sensitivity and specificity for detecting a depressive episode in adolescents, and which is included in the recommendations of the US Preventive Services Task Force, is the Patient Health Questionnaire-9 (PHQ-9) in its adolescent version (Allgaier et al., 2012; Richardson et al., 2010; US Preventive Services Task Force, 2009). The PHQ-9, being self-administered, can be used in primary healthcare, optimizing the evaluation times of patients consulting at this level of care (Hamrin & Magorno, 2010). This questionnaire has been translated and validated in different languages with adequate diagnostic validity (Borghero et al., 2018).

However, research shows that depression screening alone is not sufficient to detect suicide risk, as not all youth at suicidal risk have symptoms of depression (Kemper et al., 2021). Combined screening for depression and suicidal risk has been found to detect a more significant number of at-risk youth (Horowitz et al., 2021).

A scoping review identified 22 tools for acute suicide risk assessment in children and young people (Carter et al., 2019). Among the most used are the Ask Suicide-Screening Questions (ASQ) (Horowitz et al., 2012) and the screener version of the Columbia Suicide Severity Rating Scale (C-SSRS) (Posner et al., 2011).

The ASQ is a brief and easy-to-administer screening tool designed as a youth-specific tool for medical settings (Horowitz et al., 2012). The ASQ consists of four initial questions to assess suicidal ideation and suicidal behaviors. A "yes" or no response to any of these questions results in a positive score for suicidal risk and triggers a fifth question to assess severity. Studies show that the ASQ has high sensitivity and specificity and detects patients at risk for suicide who are not identified by depression screening alone (Horowitz et al., 2012).

The C-SSRS in its screener version for the measurement of suicidal thoughts and behaviors in youth aged 6 years and older unless it was deemed inappropriate (e.g., due to cultural context). The measure consists of six items tracking the severity of suicidal ideation in the past month and suicidal behavior in the past 3 months. The C-SSRS is free, brief, available in multiple languages, can be used by nonmental health personnel and in different settings, and has demonstrated good internal consistency, interrater reliability, and sensitivity to change in adolescent samples (Posner et al., 2011). An international consensus on a standard set of outcome measures for childhood and youth anxiety, depression, obsessive-compulsive disorder, and posttraumatic stress disorder proposes its use (Krause et al., 2021).

Once a young person screens positive for suicide risk, a further assessment is necessary, typically conducted by a physician or mental health professional. Clinicians evaluate the risk based on the youth's self-report, input from other informants, and clinical observations (Pisani et al., 2016). The assessment should be complemented with information from family members or significant others, with the patient's consent. However, it may be conducted without consent in high-risk situations while adhering to relevant legal regulations and ethical considerations. Providers should inform patients about the involvement of significant adults and discuss confidentiality. It is recommended that clinicians have private time with the patient to explore their mental health and suicide risk before engaging family members or caregivers in the care process.

Suicide risk assessment seeks to determine the current level of risk by identifying risk and protective factors. Although there is no definitive method for predicting suicide, clinical strategies are recommended to guide appropriate interventions.

The clinical interview should include at least the following:

- Suicidal ideation: Inquire about passive (desire to die) and active (desire to carry it out) thoughts, the existence of a plan, its method, and the level of intent
- Self-harm behavior: Record previous behaviors, intent, and triggers (conflicts, isolation, financial problems)
- History and psychosocial factors: Consider psychiatric history, family support, and other relevant personal circumstances

There are assessment tools that can complement the clinical interview, such as the ASQ-Brief Suicide Safety Assessment (BSSA; http://www.nimh.nih.gov/ASQ) and the C-SSRS in its assessment version (https://cssrs.columbia.edu) (http://www.cssrs.columbia.edu/) (Busby et al., 2023).

One of the factors associated with suicidal behavior that is recommended to be explored is the feeling of entrapment in the face of unbearable situations, thoughts, or emotions. This internal or external state arises from experiences of defeat or humiliation with no apparent escape (Gilbert & Allan, 1998). In a large sample of South Korean adolescents, entrapment was strongly associated with suicidal ideation beyond the influence of depression (Park et al., 2010). To measure this, De Beurs et al. (2020) developed a brief four-item version of the Entrapment Scale that could be useful for the assessment of suicidal risk in youth.

Once the assessment is completed, the clinician should integrate the clinical information into a risk formulation that allows the development of an action plan to manage suicide risk. A distinction is made between "risk status," which compares the youth's risk to others in a specific population, and "risk level," which compares it to their baseline level or at other points (Pisani et al., 2022).

Risk formulation aims not to predict outcomes but to understand and communicate the factors behind the assessment. Available internal and external resources are identified, as well as possible changes that could influence risk, especially factors that drive suicide attempts, which are key to treatment planning. Since risk fluctuates, it is important to update assessments periodically.

This formulation facilitates communication within the treatment team and with the adolescents and their families or caregivers, allowing the development of an individualized and collaborative treatment plan (Pisani et al., 2016).

7.4 Interventions

Suicide prevention interventions aim to reduce suicide incidence and suicidal behaviors within the population. These interventions seek to address risk factors, strengthen protective factors, and provide appropriate support to individuals in vulnerable situations and suicidal risk.

From a public health approach, the interventions could be classified as universal, selective, and indicated (Bailey et al., 2023; Pirkis et al., 2024a):

- Universal interventions: Aimed at the entire population, they seek to reduce barriers to accessing mental health services, increase knowledge about suicide, and strengthen protective factors such as social support. They include psychoeducation, information about services, stigma reduction, and promotion of help-seeking.
- Selective interventions: Focus on subgroups at higher risk, such as young people with depression or victims of bullying. They include screening programs, training of "gatekeepers" (community members who regularly interact with large numbers of people and are trained to detect those at risk of suicide, provide initial support, and connect them with mental health services), and support groups.
- Indicated interventions: Target individuals with warning signs, suicidal thoughts, or previous attempts. Focus on individual or group treatment by trained professionals to reduce risk and strengthen protective factors.

The WHO (2014) recommends combining these three strategies in integrated and sustained programs to achieve a significant impact.

Preventive interventions can be implemented across various environments, not exclusively by mental health providers. Developing strategies in the contexts where young individuals operate expands the opportunity to reach them quickly.

7.4.1 Interventions in Clinical Settings

Youth suicide risk screening and assessment practices should include management strategies to address both immediate and long-term safety needs. Given the difficulty in accessing specialty mental health services and high dropout rates, primary healthcare is the setting where youth in recent suicidal crises are most likely to present. Families view their primary healthcare providers as individuals who can help in times of suicidal crisis (Ruch et al., 2024).

Although primary healthcare professionals play a key role in suicide prevention, recent studies indicate that they often lack adequate training in prevention and intervention strategies. Research shows that adequately training primary healthcare personnel can significantly reduce rates of suicide, suicide attempts, and suicidal ideation (Ruch et al., 2024).

The following will present some valuable strategies for non-mental health care teams to address suicide risk in youth.

Safety planning There is growing evidence to suggest that most suicidal crises in youth are relatively brief. Approximately 50% of 11- to 15-year-olds who died by suicide showed no signs of preplanning (Holland et al., 2017), and 24% of 13- to 34-year-olds attempted suicide in a near-lethal manner after only 5 min of deliberation (Simon et al., 2001). Given that many youths contemplate suicide for a short period, targeted interventions at these times may prevent attempts. Limiting access to lethal means and using effective methods to divert suicidal thoughts play a key role in preventing youth suicide (Monahan & Stanley, 2022).

"Do-no-harm" or "do-no-suicide" contracts were introduced more than 30 years ago. However, their empirical research on their benefits is limited. A "do-no-harm " contract is a written or verbal agreement in which the patient agrees to contact a health professional, friend, or family member before engaging in self-injurious behavior. This contract usually has a specific time frame, such as until the next treatment session. In addition, "do-no-harm" contracts do not protect the clinician from legal liability if a patient dies by suicide. There is also concern that a patient at suicide risk who falsely accepts the contract may divert the clinician's attention from appropriate precautions to minimize risk. Because of the lack of evidence and the potential for harm, using these contracts is not recommended (Melvin et al., 2023).

A valuable tool to help prevent suicidal behaviors by identifying risk factors, coping strategies, and sources of support is to establish a safety plan (Stanley & Brown, 2012). A safety plan is a prioritized written list that youth can use before, during, and after a suicidal crisis. To ensure their effectiveness, plans should be developed collaboratively, involving the young people and their caregivers. The plan should be brief, readable, and in the youth's own words. It is also important to consider designing specific safety plans for the home and educational institutions, tailored to the circumstances of each setting (Monahan & Stanley, 2022).

A crucial component of this plan is counseling youth and their caregivers on how to limit access to potentially dangerous means, such as storing medications in safe places. This approach is critical in gun households, as youth in these households are at significantly increased risk for suicide (Monahan & Stanley, 2022).

In the written list, the first step is for the young person to be able to identify the warning signs that indicate an impending crisis. The second step is engaging in activities they can do autonomously to distract and calm themselves, such as listening to music or exercising. The third step encourages involving another person in activities that can help divert attention from suicidal thoughts, like watching a movie or taking a walk together. Visiting a safe public place could be recommended if social contacts are unavailable. The fourth step is to identify supportive individuals, such as family and friends, with whom the patient can discuss their suicidal thoughts. This support can help prevent the situation from escalating. The fifth step involves reaching out to a clinician for guidance or support. Additionally, the sixth step suggests calling a crisis hotline or going to an emergency department for immediate assistance (Stanley & Brown, 2012).

Some versions of the plan also include avoiding situations that they know may trigger painful memories or negative emotions and documenting reasons for living, which, when remembered, can counteract reasons for dying (Melvin et al., 2023).

It is important to note that these steps are not necessarily consecutive when using the plan is important. For example, a young person who identifies signs of impending crisis (step 1) might prefer to directly ask his or her mother for support in de-escalating suicidal thoughts (step 4), skipping steps 2 and 3.

Followup and continuity of care Unlike intensive interventions that require mental health specialists, followups are brief and inexpensive and can be delivered by trained staff on a set schedule. Although there are few clinical trials of these interventions, research suggests that they reduce repeat suicide attempts and prevent deaths after hospital discharge. Effective strategies include sending letters of support, crisis cards, and post-discharge phone contacts (Rengasamy & Sparks, 2019). In addition, ensuring that youth at risk for suicide receive a continuum of care as they transition from one healthcare setting to another is critical to saving lives and reducing suicide attempts (Sale et al., 2022)

Collaborative care models Collaborative care models in primary healthcare are increasingly recognized as practical approaches to addressing suicide risk because of their integrated, team-based approach that improves mental health care. These models are system-level interventions reorganizing healthcare delivery by connecting primary healthcare clinicians and patients with mental health specialists to provide evidence-based treatments (Goodrich et al., 2013).

Care managers are key in coordinating interventions, supporting decision-making and communication between the patient and the healthcare team, monitoring mental health symptoms and medication use, and ensuring treatment adherence (Goodrich et al., 2013).

Although there is no specific evidence on the efficacy of these models in youth at risk for suicide, they are promising interventions. Randomized clinical trials in adolescents receiving primary healthcare have demonstrated that collaborative care models are effective in reducing depression and improving adherence to evidence-based treatments (Richardson et al., 2014). In addition, family intervention, including education and improved communication, is critical to the success of interventions with youth.

7.4.2 Interventions in Community Settings

Educational settings High schools and college campuses are potential sites for targeted suicide prevention, as this setting offers continuous and direct access to a clearly defined vulnerable population, facilitating an evidence-based approach to youth suicide prevention. In addition, adolescents and young adults spend significant time in these settings, providing opportunities to implement targeted, cost-effective, and sustained interventions (Breet et al., 2021; Robinson et al., 2018).

A review of 17 studies on suicide prevention in school settings and 4 in universities found that 70% of school-based studies and 50% of university-based studies reported positive effects on reducing suicidal thoughts and behaviors. Most school-based trials focused on psychoeducation, social support, and skill-building interventions delivered by school counselors. In universities, a brief problem-solving intervention yielded positive results. Although these findings are promising, they should be interpreted cautiously due to variability in study quality. Moreover, the larger volume of research conducted in schools than universities underscores the need to address this gap in future studies (Robinson et al., 2018).

A review of 43 studies of suicide prevention interventions on educational campuses conducted primarily in high-income countries found that most interventions focused on selective strategies, with little attention to universal or indicated interventions. The studies assessed nonfatal suicidal behaviors, staff and student capacity to intervene, and knowledge about suicide but did not include suicide deaths or ecosystemic interventions. Study quality was low, with small samples and risks of bias (Breet et al., 2021).

Gatekeeper training is one of the most common suicide prevention strategies on campuses. This strategy is beneficial in resource-poor settings, where mental health professionals are scarce for timely detection and establishing early safety measures. However, ensuring timely care in the healthcare system for those who require it is also important. The authors suggest the need for more high-quality studies, especially in resource-limited countries, to evaluate interventions targeting vulnerable populations, such as LGBTQ+ youth, and to develop and test digital interventions in schools and universities, which could be an efficient and feasible way to scale up suicide prevention on campuses (Breet et al., 2021).

Community clusters Suicide can manifest in clusters, which are defined as non-random increases in suicidal behaviors in temporal or geographic proximity. Their occurrence is more common in young people (Hawton et al., 2020). A key factor in the emergence of clusters is social transmission, where one person's suicidal behavior increases the likelihood of similar behaviors in others through direct or indirect contact.

Studies have demonstrated increased suicide rates following the highly publicized deaths of celebrities, particularly among women and young people. Fictional portrayals of suicides in media series such as "13 Reasons Why" have also shown adverse effects (Sinyor et al., 2022). However, media narratives focusing on recovery may have protective effects; for example, in South Korea, suicide rates decreased after preventive laws and media guidelines (Jang et al., 2022).
The contagion effect has been the most studied mechanism underlying clusters. The "Werther effect" (Phillips, 1974) describes social transmission following media-exposed suicides, and the "Papageno effect" occurs when the media promote coping strategies and messages of hope (Niederkrotrotenthaler et al., 2010)

In the event of a cluster detection, community response is crucial. Priority must be given to identifying, evaluating, and referring individuals at the highest risk, including those close to the deceased and individuals with lived suicide experience, along with increasing the availability of mental health services and psychosocial support across community points (Ivey-Stephenson et al., 2024). Recommended interventions include psychosocial interventions, public policy regulations, and content warnings that incorporate the underlying mechanisms of these effects (Martínez et al., 2023).

Effective communication management, including safe communication protocols and avoiding sensationalism and glorification, is critical for preventing social transmission and cluster intervention (American Psychological Association 2018; Public Health of Canada 2018). This encompasses communication through media coverage, social media, internal communications, and community activities (Hill & Robinson, 2022).

Post-intervention strategies following a suicide, targeted at groups identified as most vulnerable to transmission, represent a method to minimize related suicide occurrences while simultaneously addressing the needs of bereaved individuals (Pirkis et al., 2024a, 2024b).

7.4.3 The Potential of Digital Technologies

Frequent use of social media and the Internet has been associated with suicidal behavior in young people. Social isolation, unfavorable comparisons, suicidal contagion effects, and cyberbullying may be some of the explanations for this. However, it has also been found to use positive ways to find support (Ruch et al., 2024).

Digital technologies can be an opportunity to address the barriers that prevent the timely assessment and management of suicide risk in young people (Musiat et al., 2022). Given the widespread availability of Internet access among youth, digital screening, assessment, and early intervention strategies offer a practical alternative for people at risk of suicide while overcoming some structural and attitudinal barriers to help-seeking (Ebert et al., 2019).

Programs based on digital technologies are easily accessible and scalable, allowing flexible use of available resources without time or location restrictions. Additionally, they offer high anonymity and privacy, which helps reduce the stigma and shame associated with seeking mental health support (Jiménez-Molina et al., 2019).

A potential use of technologies is to detect young people with suicide risk factors through universal screening and connect them with support services. Hasking et al. (2024) propose a promising prevention program called COMPAS-S, which uses a suicide risk algorithm embedded within a universal screening survey for university students. The COMPAS-S prevention program employed a predictive algorithm embedded within the World Mental Health International College Student (WMH-ICS) Initiative survey to identify students at higher risk of planning or attempting suicide within the next 12 months in real time. A stepped-care approach was implemented: all students received a list of local and national support services; those reporting suicidal ideation in the past 12 months were directed to a mobile safety planning application. Students flagged as high risk by the algorithm, as well as those reporting past-year suicide attempts but not identified by the algorithm, were contacted by a mental health professional within 24 h of completing the survey. The telehealth intervention focused on providing support, developing safety plans, and offering personalized referrals to appropriate services.

Another potential use of technologies is to offer internet-delivered interventions. A systematic review and meta-analysis, which includes two interventions targeting adolescents, concludes that Internet-based cognitive behavioral therapy (CBT) helps reduce suicidal ideation, but further research is needed to evaluate its impact on suicidal behaviors (Büscher et al., 2020).

One research developed the LEAP intervention, a web-based, selective preventive suicide intervention targeting adolescents' perceptions of burdensomeness toward others, based on the Interpersonal Psychological Theory of Suicide. In a pilot randomized controlled trial, results suggest that LEAP can reduce perceived burdensomeness in adolescents. The authors propose that further research is needed to improve engagement and completion rates (Hill & Pettit, 2019).

The Reframe-IT intervention is a 10-week CBT-based program for school students consisting of eight modules targeting suicidal thinking and behaviors. Participants accessed a personalized, secure web page managed by school well-being staff. After completing each module at school, students could access the content from home anytime. Modules covered emotional recognition, distress tolerance, problem-solving, and cognitive restructuring. The content was delivered through video diaries featuring young people and guided by an adult host explaining CBT concepts. Each module included two interactive activities reviewed by a clinical psychologist, who provided personalized feedback through a message board. Additional resources included fact sheets on managing suicidal thoughts and relaxation MP3s, ensuring comprehensive support while maintaining privacy and accessibility. The Reframe-IT trial faced recruitment challenges due to complex safety procedures, resulting in limited statistical power. While no significant differences were found between groups, participants engaged well with the program, showing reduced suicidal ideation, symptom improvement, and enhanced CBT skills. Notably, it was the first international online intervention trial involving youth across all suicide risk levels (Hetrick et al., 2017). One of the problems with this type of intervention is low adherence. Therefore, a blended intervention that integrates online and face-to-face components in a treatment process could address this issue. A team from Chile testing a blended intervention for adolescents, with the Internet component corresponding to REFRAME-IT, found a significant reduction in suicidal ideation (Núñez et al., 2022, 2024).

The use of this type of intervention in the field of suicide prevention is increasing and has shown promising results. However, studies among adolescents with more rigorous randomized controlled trials, including different control groups to assess the effectiveness of these interventions, are still scarce (Siadat et al., 2024). When conducting these studies with digital technologies, it is important to consider certain ethical aspects. A Consensus Statement on Ethical and Safety Practices for Conducting Digital Monitoring Studies with People at Risk of Suicide and Related Behaviors proposes specific guidelines for both the safety of participants and their sensitive data (Nock et al., 2021)

7.5 Barriers to Accessing Mental Health Care

Several studies demonstrate the effectiveness of mental health interventions in reducing the risk of suicidal behaviors among young people (Calati et al., 2018; Hughes et al., 2023; Torralba-Suarez & Olry-de-Labry-Lima, 2024). However, only 25–50% of those who report suicidal ideation or behavior seek professional help (Bruffaerts et al., 2019; Hom et al., 2015; Michelmore & Hindley, 2012). Improving access to care remains a persistent challenge in the field of mental health, underscoring the importance of identifying and addressing the barriers that limit access to interventions.

7.5.1 Structural Barriers

Structural barriers often impede young people from seeking professional mental health help support. Some of them are geographic distance to care facilities, limited availability of services, the time required for appointments, the cost of consultations and travel, and the limited knowledge about available services (Czyz et al., 2013; Downs & Eisenberg, 2012; Ebert et al., 2019; Hom et al., 2015).

For adolescents, parents frequently play a critical role in initiating and supporting mental health care. Interviews with parents of adolescents who die by suicide revealed that financial difficulties, transportation challenges, long waiting times, and lack of clarity about where to seek help were significant barriers to timely access to mental health care for their songs (Moskos et al., 2007).

Potential strategies to overcome these challenges include expanding outreach and information dissemination about available services, expanding coverage, offering extended hours, and incorporating digital technologies to facilitate access.

7.5.2 Attitudinal Barriers

While structural barriers are relevant, attitudinal and cultural factors remain the primary in accessing mental health services (Corrigan, 2004; Downs & Eisenberg, 2012; Ebert et al., 2019). These barriers exist at individual, societal, and healthcare provider levels.

Young individuals at risk of suicide often believe they can manage their problems on their own or prefer to turn to their nearby support network (Czyz et al., 2013; Downs & Eisenberg, 2012). Many fail to recognize their experiences as mental health issues requiring professional intervention or consider their symptoms insufficiently severe to seek help (Ebert et al., 2019). College students who identify as male report lower rates of perceived need for treatment (Pei et al., 2024).

Other common attitudinal barriers include the belief that treatment may not be helpful or practical, distrust of mental health professionals, concerns about confidentiality, and fear of hospitalization (Bruffaerts et al., 2011; Czyz et al., 2013; Rowe et al., 2014). Research also indicates that adolescents with severe suicidal ideation seek help to a lesser extent than those with less intense ideation (Hom et al., 2015). Although this may seem contradictory, these findings are consistent with the "help negation" concept proposed by Clark and Fawcett (1992). This term describes the process by which people with acute suicidal ideation reject available support or treatment, which is related, in part, to the hopelessness, pessimism, and maladaptive coping styles that are characteristic of people at risk for suicide (Rudd et al., 1995). Suicidal ideation itself may make it challenging to use social problem-solving skills or to employ strategies such as help-seeking (Deane et al., 2001).

Attitudinal barriers to seeking help for suicidal risk are strongly influenced by the stigma surrounding mental health, which is rooted in complex social processes.

Stigma involves labeling, stereotyping, isolating, distancing, and excluding individuals perceived as different or deviating from societal norms (Corrigan, 2004). It manifests in two key forms: perceived public stigma and personal stigma. Perceived public stigma refers to beliefs about the negative attitudes held by others toward mental health issues, while personal stigma, or self-stigma, involves an individual's negative attitudes about seeking help (Corrigan, 2004; Corrigan & Watson, 2002).

The stigma surrounding mental health remains a pervasive barrier, deeply rooted in complex social processes. Stigma manifests in two key forms: public stigma and self-stigma. Public stigma refers to negative societal attitudes toward mental health issues, while self-stigma involves an individual's internalized negative beliefs about seeking help. Although traditionally considered a significant barrier, some studies challenge its prominence. For instance, only 12% reported stigma as a barrier to care (Czyz et al., 2013). Nonetheless, stigma should not be overlooked. Public stigma remains prevalent, as many at-risk youths fear adverse reactions from others and are being labeled as "just looking for attention" (Rowe et al., 2014). On the other hand, some youth exhibit personal stigma, viewing acknowledging the need for mental health help as a sign of weakness, incompetence, or personal failure (Vidourek et al., 2014). Other barriers to care reported by a significant proportion of youth at suicidal risks, such as lack of perceived need, may capture more subtle aspects of stigma (Hom et al., 2015).

Stigma may disproportionately affect specific groups, including the LGBT+ population (Crockett et al., 2022), racial and ethnic minoritized groups, and men (Pei et al., 2024). Educational settings represent a key opportunity to implement interventions that address mental health stigma. These actions can be complemented with anti-stigma campaigns targeting specific populations, such as those previously mentioned, as well as other groups, including men and migrants with depression (Martinez et al., 2020).

In a recent systematic review and meta-analysis of 97 randomized clinical trials, anti-stigma interventions generated small to moderately significant improvements in mental health stigma-related knowledge, attitudes, behaviors, and general stigma. In addition, minimal but significant improvements were observed in attitudes and help-seeking intentions. However, these effects diminish, highlighting the need for ongoing work to sustain such improvements (Crockett et al., 2025).

Attitudinal barriers can be addressed through appropriate psychoeducation to recognize when faced with a mental health problem that requires professional help. This approach should be directed at both youth at risk of suicide and their close environment, encouraging early detection and timely support-seeking.

7.6 Future Directions

Early identification and timely intervention for youth suicide risk is a global imperative.

Understanding how intersecting social identities—such as race, gender identity, and socioeconomic status—influence suicide risk and protective factors is crucial to developing culturally sensitive and inclusive prevention programs. Longitudinal research is needed to track the evolution of these risk and protective factors across adolescence and young adulthood.

Suicide risk assessment tools should be refined for diverse linguistic and cultural populations. In addition, studies should compare the long-term efficacy of universal versus targeted screening methods. Expanding screening efforts to schools, community centers, and digital platforms could reach at-risk youth who do not seek medical care.

The rise of digital platforms presents new opportunities for suicide prevention. artificial intelligence (AI) and machine learning offer promising avenues. Research should explore the role of social networks, mobile apps, and online counseling in providing timely support. Interactive digital interventions, such as gamification and virtual reality, could improve engagement and adherence. It is essential to strengthen ethical guidelines and policies to safeguard data privacy and participant safety.

It is crucial to train primary care providers in suicide risk assessment and intervention, foster collaborative care models, ensure continuity of care, and implement hybrid care approaches that integrate in-person and virtual support to address accessibility barriers.

Crisis intervention strategies for people with acute mental disorders, as well as postvention efforts for suicide survivors and affected communities, should be further examined.

Culturally tailored prevention strategies are especially vital in low- and middle-income countries, where resource scarcity and stigma pose significant barriers.

Community-based initiatives require rigorous evaluation, including peer support programs and mental health awareness campaigns.

Policy strategies must also address the social determinants of health, such as poverty, discrimination, and accessibility of health care. Financing policies should ensure affordable mental health services and universal coverage.

Acknowledgments This manuscript was supported by ANID—Millennium Science Initiative Program—AIM23_0002 and NCS2021_081 and by ANID—Fondecyt Project N° 1221230. BV received funding from ANID/BECA DOCTORADO NACIONAL/2021_21212114.

References

Allgaier, A. K., Pietsch, K., Frühe, B., Sigl-Glöckner, J., & Schulte-Körne, G. (2012). Screening for depression in adolescents: Validity of the patient health questionnaire in pediatric care. *Depression and Anxiety, 29*(10), 906–913. https://doi.org/10.1002/da.21971

American Academy of Pediatrics. (2022). *Suicide: Blueprint for youth suicide prevention.* Accessed November 04, 2024, from https://www.aap.org/suicideprevention

American Psychological Association. (2018). *APA dictionary of psychology*. Accessed November 04, 2024, from https://dictionary.apa.org/social-contagion

Bauer, G. R., Churchill, S. M., Mahendran, M., Walwyn, C., Lizotte, D., & Villa-Rueda, A. A. (2021). Intersectionality in quantitative research: A systematic review of its emergence and applications of theory and methods. *SSM – Population Health, 14*, 100798. https://doi.org/10.1016/j.ssmph.2021.100798

Bailey, E., Robinson, J., & Witt, K. (2023). Interventions for youth suicide and suicide-related behaviour: An update to a systematic review. *Australasian Psychiatry, 31*(4), 505–523. https://doi.org/10.1177/10398562231187972

Bakken, V., Lydersen, S., Skokauskas, N., Sund, A. M., & Kaasbøll, J. (2024). Protective factors for suicidal ideation: A prospective study from adolescence to adulthood. *European Child & Adolescent Psychiatry, 33*(9), 3079–3089. https://doi.org/10.1007/s00787-024-02379-w

Borghero, F., Martínez, V., Zitko, P., Vöhringer, P. A., Cavada, G., & Rojas, G. (2018). Tamizaje de episodio depresivo en adolescentes. Validación del instrumento PHQ-9 [Screening depressive episodes in adolescents. Validation of the Patient Health Questionnaire-9 (PHQ-9)]. *Revista medica de Chile, 146*(4), 479–486. https://doi.org/10.4067/s0034-98872018000400479

Breet, E., Matooane, M., Tomlinson, M., & Bantjes, J. (2021). Systematic review and narrative synthesis of suicide prevention in high-schools and universities: A research agenda for evidence-based practice. *BMC Public Health, 21*(1), 1116. https://doi.org/10.1186/s12889-021-11124-w

Bruffaerts, R., Demyttenaere, K., Hwang, I., Chiu, W. T., Sampson, N., Kessler, R. C., Alonso, J., Borges, G., de Girolamo, G., de Graaf, R., Florescu, S., Gureje, O., Hu, C., Karam, E. G., Kawakami, N., Kostyuchenko, S., Kovess-Masfety, V., Lee, S., Levinson, D., Matschinger, H., … Nock, M. K. (2011). Treatment of suicidal people around the world. The British journal of psychiatry: the journal of mental science, 199(1), 64–70. https://doi.org/10.1192/bjp.bp.110.084129

Bruffaerts, R., Mortier, P., Auerbach, R. P., Alonso, J., Hermosillo De la Torre, A. E., Cuijpers, P., Demyttenaere, K., Ebert, D. D., Green, J. G., Hasking, P., Stein, D. J., Ennis, E., Nock, M. K., Pinder-Amaker, S., Sampson, N. A., Vilagut, G., Zaslavsky, A. M., Kessler, R. C., & WHO WMH-ICS Collaborators. (2019). Lifetime and 12-month treatment for mental disorders and suicidal thoughts and behaviors among first year college students. *International Journal of Methods in Psychiatric Research, 28*(2), e1764. https://doi.org/10.1002/mpr.1764

Busby, D. R., Hughes, J. L., Walters, M., Ihediwa, A., Adeniran, M., Goodman, L., & Mayes, T. L. (2023). Measurement choices for youth suicidality. *Child Psychiatry and Human Development*. Advance online publication. https://doi.org/10.1007/s10578-023-01627-5

Büscher, R., Torok, M., Terhorst, Y., & Sander, L. (2020). Internet-based cognitive behavioral therapy to reduce suicidal ideation: A systematic review and meta-analysis. *JAMA Network Open, 3*(4), e203933. https://doi.org/10.1001/jamanetworkopen.2020.3933

Calati, R., Courtet, P., & Lopez-Castroman, J. (2018). Refining suicide prevention: A narrative review on advances in psychotherapeutic tools. *Current Psychiatry Reports, 20*(2), 14. https://doi.org/10.1007/s11920-018-0876-0

Cantor, N., Kingsbury, M., Warner, E., Landry, H., Clayborne, Z., Islam, R., & Colman, I. (2023). Young adult outcomes associated with adolescent suicidality: A meta-analysis. *Pediatrics, 151*(3), e2022058113. https://doi.org/10.1542/peds.2022-058113

Carter, T., Walker, G. M., Aubeeluck, A., & Manning, J. C. (2019). Assessment tools of immediate risk of self-harm and suicide in children and young people: A scoping review. *Journal of Child Health Care for Professionals Working with Children in the Hospital and Community, 23*(2), 178–199. https://doi.org/10.1177/1367493518787925

Clark, D. C., & Fawcett, J. B. (1992). Review of empirical risk factors for evaluation of the suicidal patient. In B. M. Bongar (Ed.), *Suicide: Guidelines for assessment, management, and treatment* (pp. 16–48). Oxford University Press.

Corrigan, P. (2004). How stigma interferes with mental health care. *The American Psychologist, 59*(7), 614–625. https://doi.org/10.1037/0003-066X.59.7.614

Corrigan, P. W., & Watson, A. C. (2002). Understanding the impact of stigma on people with mental illness. *World Psychiatry, 1*(1), 16–20.

Crockett, M. A., Martínez, V., & Caviedes, P. (2022). Barriers and facilitators to mental health help-seeking and experiences with service use among LGBT+ university students in Chile. *International Journal of Environmental Research and Public Health, 19*(24), 16520. https://doi.org/10.3390/ijerph192416520

Crockett, M. A., Núñez, D., Martínez, P., Borghero, F., Campos, S., Langer, Á. I., Carrasco, J., & Martínez, V. (2025). Interventions to reduce mental health stigma in young people: A systematic review and meta-analysis. *JAMA Network Open, 8*(1), e2454730. https://doi.org/10.1001/jamanetworkopen.2024.54730

Czyz, E. K., Horwitz, A. G., Eisenberg, D., Kramer, A., & King, C. A. (2013). Self-reported barriers to professional help seeking among college students at elevated risk for suicide. *Journal of American College Health, 61*(7), 398–406. https://doi.org/10.1080/07448481.2013.820731

De Beurs, D., Cleare, S., Wetherall, K., Eschle-Byrne, S., Ferguson, E., O'Connor, B., & O'Connor, R. (2020). Entrapment and suicide risk: The development of the 4-item Entrapment Scale Short-Form (E-SF). *Psychiatry Research, 284*, 112765. https://doi.org/10.1016/j.psychres.2020.112765

Deane, F. P., Wilson, C. J., & Ciarrochi, J. (2001). Suicidal ideation and help-negation: Not just hopelessness or prior help. *Journal of Clinical Psychology, 57*(7), 901–914. https://doi.org/10.1002/jclp.1058

Downs, M. F., & Eisenberg, D. (2012). Help seeking and treatment use among suicidal college students. *Journal of American College Health, 60*(2), 104–114. https://doi.org/10.1080/07448481.2011.619611

Ebert, D. D., Mortier, P., Kaehlke, F., Bruffaerts, R., Baumeister, H., Auerbach, R. P., Alonso, J., Vilagut, G., Martínez, K. I., Lochner, C., Cuijpers, P., Kuechler, A. M., Green, J., Hasking, P., Lapsley, C., Sampson, N. A., Kessler, R. C., & WHO World Mental Health-International College Student Initiative collaborators. (2019). Barriers of mental health treatment utilization among first-year college students: First cross-national results from the WHO World Mental Health International College Student Initiative. *International Journal of Methods in Psychiatric Research, 28*(2), e1782. https://doi.org/10.1002/mpr.1782

Franklin, J. C., Ribeiro, J. D., Fox, K. R., Bentley, K. H., Kleiman, E. M., Huang, X., Musacchio, K. M., Jaroszewski, A. C., Chang, B. P., & Nock, M. K. (2017). Risk factors for suicidal thoughts and behaviors: A meta-analysis of 50 years of research. *Psychological Bulletin, 143*(2), 187–232. https://doi.org/10.1037/bul0000084

Gilbert, P., & Allan, S. (1998). The role of defeat and entrapment (arrested flight) in depression: An exploration of an evolutionary view. *Psychological Medicine, 28*(3), 585–598. https://doi.org/10.1017/s0033291798006710

Goto, R., Okubo, Y., & Skokauskas, N. (2022). Reasons and trends in youth's suicide rates during the COVID-19 pandemic. *The Lancet Regional Health. Western Pacific, 27*, 100567. https://doi.org/10.1016/j.lanwpc.2022.100567

Goodrich, D. E., Kilbourne, A. M., Nord, K. M., & Bauer, M. S. (2013). Mental health collaborative care and its role in primary care settings. *Current Psychiatry Reports, 15*(8), 383. https://doi.org/10.1007/s11920-013-0383-2

Hamrin, V., & Magorno, M. (2010). Assessment of adolescents for depression in the pediatric primary care setting. *Pediatric Nursing, 36*(2), 103–111.

Hasking, P. A., Robinson, K., McEvoy, P., Melvin, G., Bruffaerts, R., Boyes, M. E., Auerbach, R. P., Hendrie, D., Nock, M. K., Preece, D. A., Rees, C., & Kessler, R. C. (2024). Development and evaluation of a predictive algorithm and telehealth intervention to reduce suicidal behavior among university students. *Psychological medicine, 54*(5), 971–979. https://doi.org/10.1017/S0033291723002714.

Hawton, K., Hill, N. T. M., Gould, M., John, A., Lascelles, K., & Robinson, J. (2020). Clustering of suicides in children and adolescents. *The Lancet. Child & Adolescent Health, 4*(1), 58–67. https://doi.org/10.1016/S2352-4642(19)30335-9

Hawton, K., Lascelles, K., Pitman, A., Gilbert, S., & Silverman, M. (2022). Assessment of suicide risk in mental health practice: Shifting from prediction to therapeutic assessment, formulation, and risk management. *The Lancet. Psychiatry, 9*(11), 922–928. https://doi.org/10.1016/S2215-0366(22)00232-2

Hetrick, S. E., Yuen, H. P., Bailey, E., Cox, G. R., Templer, K., Rice, S. M., Bendall, S., & Robinson, J. (2017). Internet-based cognitive behavioural therapy for young people with suicide-related behaviour (Reframe-IT): A randomised controlled trial. *Evidence-Based Mental Health, 20*(3), 76–82. https://doi.org/10.1136/eb-2017-102719

Hill, R. M., & Pettit, J. W. (2019). Pilot randomized controlled trial of LEAP: A selective preventive intervention to reduce adolescents' perceived burdensomeness. *Journal of Clinical Child and Adolescent Psychology, 48*(Suppl 1), S45–S56. https://doi.org/10.1080/15374416.2016.1188705

Hill, N. T. M., & Robinson, J. (2022). Responding to suicide clusters in the community: What do existing suicide cluster response frameworks recommend and how are they implemented? *International Journal of Environmental Research and Public Health, 19*(8), 4444. https://doi.org/10.3390/ijerph19084444

Holland, K. M., Vivolo-Kantor, A. M., Logan, J. E., & Leemis, R. W. (2017). Antecedents of suicide among youth aged 11–15: A multistate mixed methods analysis. *Journal of Youth and Adolescence, 46*(7), 1598–1610. https://doi.org/10.1007/s10964-016-0610-3

Hom, M. A., Stanley, I. H., & Joiner, T. E., Jr. (2015). Evaluating factors and interventions that influence help-seeking and mental health service utilization among suicidal individuals: A review of the literature. *Clinical Psychology Review, 40*, 28–39. https://doi.org/10.1016/j.cpr.2015.05.006

Horowitz, L. M., Bridge, J. A., Teach, S. J., Ballard, E., Klima, J., Rosenstein, D. L., Wharff, E. A., Ginnis, K., Cannon, E., Joshi, P., & Pao, M. (2012). Ask suicide-screening questions (ASQ): A brief instrument for the pediatric emergency department. *Archives of Pediatrics & Adolescent Medicine, 166*(12), 1170–1176. https://doi.org/10.1001/archpediatrics.2012.1276

Horowitz, L. M., Mournet, A. M., Lanzillo, E., He, J. P., Powell, D. S., Ross, A. M., Wharff, E. A., Bridge, J. A., & Pao, M. (2021). Screening pediatric medical patients for suicide risk: Is depression screening enough? *The Journal of Adolescent Health, 68*(6), 1183–1188. https://doi.org/10.1016/j.jadohealth.2021.01.028

Hughes, J. L., Horowitz, L. M., Ackerman, J. P., Adrian, M. C., Campo, J. V., & Bridge, J. A. (2023). Suicide in young people: Screening, risk assessment, and intervention. *BMJ (Clinical Research Ed.), 381*, e070630. https://doi.org/10.1136/bmj-2022-070630

Ivey-Stephenson, A. Z., Ballesteros, M. F., Trinh, E., Stone, D. M., & Crosby, A. E. (2024). CDC guidance for community response to suicide clusters, United States, 2024. *MMWR Supplements, 73*(2), 17–26. https://doi.org/10.15585/mmwr.su7302a3

Jang, J., Myung, W., Kim, S., Han, M., Yook, V., Kim, E. J., & Jeon, H. J. (2022). Effect of suicide prevention law and media guidelines on copycat suicide of general population following celebrity suicides in South Korea, 2005-2017. *The Australian and New Zealand Journal of Psychiatry, 56*(5), 542–550. https://doi.org/10.1177/00048674211025701

Jiménez-Molina, Á., Franco, P., Martínez, V., Martínez, P., Rojas, G., & Araya, R. (2019). Internet-based interventions for the prevention and treatment of mental disorders in Latin America: A scoping review. *Frontiers in Psychiatry, 10*, 664. https://doi.org/10.3389/fpsyt.2019.00664

Kemper, A. R., Hostutler, C. A., Beck, K., Fontanella, C. A., & Bridge, J. A. (2021). Depression and suicide-risk screening results in pediatric primary care. *Pediatrics, 148*(1), e2021049999. https://doi.org/10.1542/peds.2021-049999

Kim, S., Park, J., Lee, H., Lee, H., Woo, S., Kwon, R., Kim, S., Koyanagi, A., Smith, L., Rahmati, M., Fond, G., Boyer, L., Kang, J., Lee, J. H., Oh, J., & Yon, D. K. (2024). Global public concern of childhood and adolescence suicide: A new perspective and new strategies for suicide prevention in the post-pandemic era. *World Journal of Pediatrics, 20*(9), 872–900. https://doi.org/10.1007/s12519-024-00828-9

Krause, K. R., Chung, S., Adewuya, A. O., Albano, A. M., Babins-Wagner, R., Birkinshaw, L., Brann, P., Creswell, C., Delaney, K., Falissard, B., Forrest, C. B., Hudson, J. L., Ishikawa, S. I., Khatwani, M., Kieling, C., Krause, J., Malik, K., Martínez, V., Mughal, F., Ollendick, T. H., et al. (2021). International consensus on a standard set of outcome measures for child and youth anxiety, depression, obsessive-compulsive disorder, and post-traumatic stress disorder. *The Lancet Psychiatry, 8*(1), 76–86. https://doi.org/10.1016/S2215-0366(20)30356-4

Lund, C., Brooke-Sumner, C., Baingana, F., Baron, E. C., Breuer, E., Chandra, P., Haushofer, J., Herrman, H., Jordans, M., Kieling, C., Medina-Mora, M. E., Morgan, E., Omigbodun, O., Tol, W., Patel, V., & Saxena, S. (2018). Social determinants of mental disorders and the Sustainable Development Goals: A systematic review of reviews. *The Lancet. Psychiatry, 5*(4), 357–369. https://doi.org/10.1016/S2215-0366(18)30060-9

Maciá-Casas, A., de la Iglesia-Larrad, J., García-Ullán, L., Refoyo-Matellán, B., Munaiz-Cossío, C., Díaz-Trejo, S., Berdión-Marcos, V., Calama-Martín, J., Roncero, C., & Pérez, J. (2024). Post-pandemic evolution of suicide risk in children and adolescents attending a general hospital accident and emergency department. *Healthcare (Basel, Switzerland), 12*(10), 977. https://doi.org/10.3390/healthcare12100977

Marmot, M., Friel, S., Bell, R., Houweling, T. A. J., Taylor, S., & Commission social determinants, H. (2008). Closing the gap in a generation: Health equity through action on the social determinants of health. *Lancet, 372*(9650), 1661–1669. https://doi.org/10.1016/s0140-6736(08)61690-6

Martínez, V., Crockett, M. A., Jiménez-Molina, Á., Espinosa-Duque, H. D., Barrientos, E., & Ordóñez-Carrasco, J. L. (2020). Stigmatizing beliefs and attitudes to depression in adolescent school students in Chile and Colombia. *Frontiers in Psychology, 11*, 577177. https://doi.org/10.3389/fpsyg.2020.577177

Martínez, V., Jiménez-Molina, Á., & Gerber, M. M. (2023). Social contagion, violence, and suicide among adolescents. *Current Opinion in Psychiatry, 36*(3), 237–242. https://doi.org/10.1097/YCO.0000000000000858

Mathias, C. W., Michael Furr, R., Sheftall, A. H., Hill-Kapturczak, N., Crum, P., & Dougherty, D. M. (2012). What's the harm in asking about suicidal ideation? *Suicide & Life-Threatening Behavior, 42*(3), 341–351. https://doi.org/10.1111/j.1943-278X.2012.0095.x

Melvin, G. A., Oquendo, M. A., Stanley, B., & Posner, K. (2023). Assessment and management of suicidal risk. In *Tasman's Psychiatry* (pp. 1–32). Springer International. https://doi.org/10.1007/978-3-030-42825-9_67-1

Michelmore, L., & Hindley, P. (2012). Help-seeking for suicidal thoughts and self-harm in young people: A systematic review. *Suicide & Life-Threatening Behavior, 42*(5), 507–524. https://doi.org/10.1111/j.1943-278X.2012.00108.x

Misiak, B., Samochowiec, J., Gawęda, Ł., & Frydecka, D. (2023). Association of sociodemographic, proximal, and distal clinical factors with current suicidal ideation: Findings from a nonclinical sample of young adults. *European Psychiatry: The Journal of the Association of European Psychiatrists, 66*(1), e29. https://doi.org/10.1192/j.eurpsy.2023.14

Monahan, M. F., & Stanley, B. (2022). Safety planning and lethal means counseling with youth. In J. P. Ackerman & L. M. Horowitz (Eds.), *Youth suicide prevention and intervention. Springerbriefs in psychology*. Springer. https://doi.org/10.1007/978-3-031-06127-1_9

Moskos, M. A., Olson, L., Halbern, S. R., & Gray, D. (2007). Utah youth suicide study: Barriers to mental health treatment for adolescents. *Suicide & Life-Threatening Behavior, 37*(2), 179–186. https://doi.org/10.1521/suli.2007.37.2.179

Musiat, P., Johnson, C., Atkinson, M., Wilksch, S., & Wade, T. (2022). Impact of guidance on intervention adherence in computerised interventions for mental health problems: A meta-analysis. *Psychological Medicine, 52*(2), 229–240. https://doi.org/10.1017/S0033291721004621

Niederkrotenthaler, T., Voracek, M., Herberth, A., Till, B., Strauss, M., Etzersdorfer, E., Eisenwort, B., & Sonneck, G. (2010). Role of media reports in completed and prevented suicide: Werther v. Papageno effects. *The British Journal of Psychiatry, 197*(3), 234–243. https://doi.org/10.1192/bjp.bp.109.074633

Na, P. J., Shin, J., Kwak, H. R., Lee, J., Jester, D. J., Bandara, P., Kim, J. Y., Moutier, C. Y., Pietrzak, R. H., Oquendo, M. A., & Jeste, D. V. (2025). Social determinants of health and suicide-related outcomes: A review of meta-analyses. *JAMA Psychiatry*. https://doi.org/10.1001/jamapsychiatry.2024.4241

Nock, M. K., Kleiman, E. M., Abraham, M., Bentley, K. H., Brent, D. A., Buonopane, R. J., Castro-Ramirez, F., Cha, C. B., Dempsey, W., Draper, J., Glenn, C. R., Harkavy-Friedman, J., Hollander, M. R., Huffman, J. C., Lee, H. I. S., Millner, A. J., Mou, D., Onnela, J. P., Picard, R. W., Quay, H. M., et al. (2021). Consensus statement on ethical & safety practices for conducting digital monitoring studies with people at risk of suicide and related behaviors. *Psychiatric Research and Clinical Practice, 3*(2), 57–66. https://doi.org/10.1176/appi.prcp.20200029

Núñez, D., Gaete, J., Meza, D., Andaur, J., & Robinson, J. (2022). Testing the effectiveness of a blended intervention to reduce suicidal ideation among school adolescents in Chile: A protocol for a cluster randomized controlled trial. *International Journal of Environmental Research and Public Health, 19*(7), 3947. https://doi.org/10.3390/ijerph19073947

Nuñez, D., Meza, D., Andaur, J., Robinson, J., & Gaete, J. (2024). Reframe-IT+, an indicated preventive school-based intervention, reduces suicidal ideation among adolescents in vulnerable contexts in Chile. *BMC Psychology, 12*(1), 780. https://doi.org/10.1186/s40359-024-02300-9

Park, Y. J., Ryu, H., Han, K., Kwon, J. H., Kim, H. K., Kang, H. C., Yoon, J. W., Cheon, S. H., & Shin, H. (2010). Suicidal ideation in adolescents: An explanatory model using LISREL. *Western Journal of Nursing Research, 32*(2), 168–184. https://doi.org/10.1177/0193945909349115

Pei, J., Amanvermez, Y., Vigo, D., Puyat, J., Kessler, R. C., Mortier, P., Bruffaerts, R., Rankin, O., Chua, S. N., Martínez, V., Rapsey, C., Fodor, L. A., David, O. A., Garcia, C., & Cuijpers, P. (2024). Sociodemographic correlates of mental health treatment seeking among college students: A systematic review and meta-analysis. *Psychiatric Services (Washington, D.C.), 75*(6), 556–569. https://doi.org/10.1176/appi.ps.20230414

Phillips, D. P. (1974). The influence of suggestion on suicide: Substantive and theoretical implications of the Werther effect. *American Sociological Review, 39*(3), 340–354.

Pirkis, J., Bantjes, J., Gould, M., Niederkrotenthaler, T., Robinson, J., Sinyor, M., Ueda, M., & Hawton, K. (2024a). Public health measures related to the transmissibility of suicide. *The Lancet Public Health, 9*(10), e807–e815. https://doi.org/10.1016/S2468-2667(24)00153-1

Pirkis, J., Dandona, R., Silverman, M., Khan, M., & Hawton, K. (2024b). Preventing suicide: A public health approach to a global problem. *The Lancet. Public health, 9*(10), e787–e795. https://doi.org/10.1016/S2468-2667(24)00149-X

Pisani, A. R., Murrie, D. C., & Silverman, M. M. (2016). Reformulating suicide risk formulation: From prediction to prevention. *Academic Psychiatry, 40*(4), 623–629. https://doi.org/10.1007/s40596-015-0434-6

Pisani, A. R., Murrie, D. C., Silverman, M., & Turner, K. (2022). Prevention-oriented risk formulation. In M. Pompili (Ed.), *Suicide risk assessment and prevention*. Springer. https://doi.org/10.1007/978-3-030-42003-1_13

Posner, K., Brown, G. K., Stanley, B., Brent, D. A., Yershova, K. V., Oquendo, M. A., Currier, G. W., Melvin, G. A., Greenhill, L., Shen, S., & Mann, J. J. (2011). The Columbia-Suicide Severity Rating Scale: Initial validity and internal consistency findings from three multisite studies with adolescents and adults. *The American Journal of Psychiatry, 168*(12), 1266–1277. https://doi.org/10.1176/appi.ajp.2011.10111704

Public Health of Canada, Centre for Suicide Prevention and l'Association québécoise de prévention du suicide. (2018). *Language Matters: Safe Communication for Suicide Prevention*. Accessed November 04, 2024, from https://www.canada.ca/en/public-health/services/publications/healthy-living/language-matters-safe-communication-suicide-prevention.html

Rengasamy, M., & Sparks, G. (2019). Reduction of postdischarge suicidal behavior among adolescents through a telephone-based intervention. *Psychiatric Services (Washington, D.C.), 70*(7), 545–552. https://doi.org/10.1176/appi.ps.201800421

Richardson, L. P., Ludman, E., McCauley, E., Lindenbaum, J., Larison, C., Zhou, C., Clarke, G., Brent, D., & Katon, W. (2014). Collaborative care for adolescents with depression in primary care: A randomized clinical trial. *JAMA, 312*(8), 809–816. https://doi.org/10.1001/jama.2014.9259

Richardson, L. P., McCauley, E., Grossman, D. C., McCarty, C. A., Richards, J., Russo, J. E., Rockhill, C., & Katon, W. (2010). Evaluation of the Patient Health Questionnaire-9 Item for detecting major depression among adolescents. *Pediatrics, 126*(6), 1117–1123. https://doi.org/10.1542/peds.2010-0852

Robinson, J., Calear, A. L., & Bailey, E. (2018). Suicide prevention in educational settings: A review. *Australasian Psychiatry: Bulletin of Royal Australian and New Zealand College of Psychiatrists, 26*(2), 132–140. https://doi.org/10.1177/1039856218759406

Rowe, S. L., French, R. S., Henderson, C., Ougrin, D., Slade, M., & Moran, P. (2014). Help-seeking behaviour and adolescent self-harm: A systematic review. *The Australian and New Zealand Journal of Psychiatry, 48*(12), 1083–1095. https://doi.org/10.1177/0004867414555718

Ruch, D. A., Hughes, J. L., Bridge, J. A., & Fontanella, C. A. (2024). Evidence-based youth suicide prevention and intervention in pediatric primary care settings. *Pediatric Clinics of North America, 71*(6), 1119–1140. https://doi.org/10.1016/j.pcl.2024.07.017

Ruch, D. A., Sheftall, A. H., Schlagbaum, P., Rausch, J., Campo, J. V., & Bridge, J. A. (2019). Trends in suicide among youth aged 10 to 19 years in the United States, 1975 to 2016. *JAMA Network Open, 2*(5), e193886. https://doi.org/10.1001/jamanetworkopen.2019.3886

Rudd, M. D., Joiner, T. E., Jr., & Rajab, M. H. (1995). Help negation after acute suicidal crisis. *Journal of Consulting and Clinical Psychology, 63*(3), 499–503. https://doi.org/10.1037/0022-006x.63.3.499

Sale, E., Sandhu, A. S., & VonDras, S. (2022). Effectiveness of a continuity-of-care model to reduce youth suicidality. *Crisis, 43*(6), 486–492. https://doi.org/10.1027/0227-5910/a000818

Salinas-Contreras, M., Vargas, B., Crockett, M. A., & Martinez, V. (2023). Disparities in the use of mental health services of adolescents in Chile. *Andes Pediatrica: Revista Chilena De Pediatria, 94*(6), 681–688. https://doi.org/10.32641/andespediatr.v94i6.4637

Siadat, S., Farajzadegan, Z., Motamedi, N., Nouri, R., & Eizadi-Mood, N. (2024). Technology-based suicide prevention: An umbrella review. *Journal of Research in Medical Sciences, 29*, 28. https://doi.org/10.4103/jrms.jrms_791_23

Simon, T. R., Swann, A. C., Powell, K. E., Potter, L. B., Kresnow, M. J., & O'Carroll, P. W. (2001). Characteristics of impulsive suicide attempts and attempters. *Suicide and Life-Threatening Behavior, 32*(1), 49–59. https://doi.org/10.1521/suli.32.1.5.49.24212

Sinyor, M., Mallia, E., de Oliveira, C., Schaffer, A., Niederkrotenthaler, T., Zaheer, J., Mitchell, R., Rudoler, D., & Kurdyak, P. (2022). Emergency department visits for self-harm in adolescents after release of the Netflix series '13 Reasons Why'. *The Australian and New Zealand Journal of Psychiatry, 56*(11), 1434–1442. https://doi.org/10.1177/00048674211065999

Stanley, B., & Brown, G. K. (2012). Safety planning intervention: A brief intervention to mitigate suicide risk. *Cognitive and Behavioral Practice, 19*(2), 256–264. https://doi.org/10.1016/j.cbpra.2011.01.001

Torralba-Suarez, C., & Olry-de-Labry-Lima, A. (2024). An umbrella review of cognitive behavioural and dialectical behavioural therapies to treat self-harm and suicidal behaviour in adolescents. *Actas espanolas de psiquiatria, 52*(4), 549–560. https://doi.org/10.62641/aep.v52i4.1631

US Preventive Services Task Force. (2009). Screening and treatment for major depressive disorder in children and adolescents: US Preventive Services Task Force Recommendation Statement. *Pediatrics, 123*(4), 1223–1228. https://doi.org/10.1542/peds.2008-2381

Vidourek, R. A., King, K. A., Nabors, L. A., & Merianos, A. L. (2014). Students' benefits and barriers to mental health help-seeking. *Health Psychology and Behavioral Medicine, 2*(1), 1009–1022. https://doi.org/10.1080/21642850.2014.963586

Wasserman, D., Carli, V., Iosue, M., Javed, A., & Herrman, H. (2021). Suicide prevention in childhood and adolescence: A narrative review of current knowledge on risk and protective factors and effectiveness of interventions. *Asia-Pacific Psychiatry, 13*(3), e12452. https://doi.org/10.1111/appy.12452

World Health Organization. (2014). *Preventing suicide: A global imperative*. Accessed November 04, 2024, from https://iris.who.int/handle/10665/131056

World Health Organization. (2024). *Suicide.* Accessed November 04, 2024, from https://www.who.int/news-room/fact-sheets/detail/suicide

World Health Organization Commission on Social Determinants of Health, & World Health Organization. (2008). *Closing the gap in a generation: Health equity through action on the social determinants of health: Commission on Social Determinants of Health final report.* World Health Organization. Accessed November 04, 2024, from https://www.who.int/publications/i/item/WHO-IER-CSDH-08.1

Chapter 8
The Role of Digital Technology in Youth Suicide Prevention

Bridget Kenny, Jo Robinson, and Daniel Núñez

8.1 Addressing Youth Suicide

Suicide is a leading cause of death for adolescents and young people globally (World Health Organization, 2021a, b), and increasing rates of suicidal thoughts and behaviors among young people have been observed in several countries (Australian Institute of Health and Welfare, 2023; Ruch et al., 2019). Youth suicide does not only represent a tragic loss of individual potential but has a significant impact on the broader community. Given the pervasive and worsening nature of youth suicide, there is an urgent need to develop innovative strategies that effectively address this issue.

Suicide prevention and early intervention strategies have historically been delivered within health services. However, many young people at risk for suicide are not engaged with health services (Walby et al., 2018) due to stigma-related concerns, shame, geographic isolation, and/or lack of knowledge about services; these barriers are often exacerbated for young people from minority groups (Brown et al., 2016; Radez et al., 2021). The availability and accessibility of appropriate services for young people is another important concern. Complicated pathways to care and long wait times present key barriers to mental health services (Anderson et al., 2017). Even in circumstances where young people are engaged with health services, they must disclose their distress or intention to harm, and evidence suggests young

B. Kenny · J. Robinson
Orygen, The Centre for Youth Mental Health, University of Melbourne, Melbourne, Australia

D. Núñez (✉)
Faculty of Psychology, Universidad de Talca, Talca, Chile

Nucleus to Improve the Mental Health of Adolescents and Youths (Imhay), Santiago, Chile
e-mail: dnunez@utalca.cl

Á. Jiménez-Molina, V. Martínez (eds.), *New Perspectives on Suicidal Behavior, Depression and Personality*, https://doi.org/10.1007/978-3-031-96037-6_8

people often refrain from disclosing suicide risk to clinicians and other adults (Osborne et al., 2023).

The rise of digital technology offers promise and may address some of the barriers inherent in current approaches (e.g., accessibility, acceptability), particularly among young people, given their high digital literacy skills. Digital technology interventions can be delivered relatively quickly to many people, including marginalized or geographically isolated (Luxton et al., 2011). They can also allow young people to access information and highly personalized support in real time, at all times of the day and night, through various devices, including smartphones, tablets, and computers (Luxton et al., 2011). Digital interventions may be accessed anonymously, which can be an incentive for young people, particularly if they experience stigma-related concerns. These technologies also offer young people the opportunity to connect with peers, either anonymously or not, who they would be otherwise unable to access; this is particularly important for young people from minority groups and/or who are geographically isolated (Selkie et al., 2020).

Digital technologies may be used to deliver universal, selective, and indicated suicide prevention interventions. Universal interventions are designed to reach all young people, regardless of their risk; selective interventions target young people who may be at risk of experiencing suicidal distress; and indicated interventions aim to support young people exhibiting early signs of suicidal distress (World Health Organization, 2014).

This chapter provides an overview of current approaches to youth suicide prevention (see Fig. 8.1), highlighting how universal, selective, and indicated

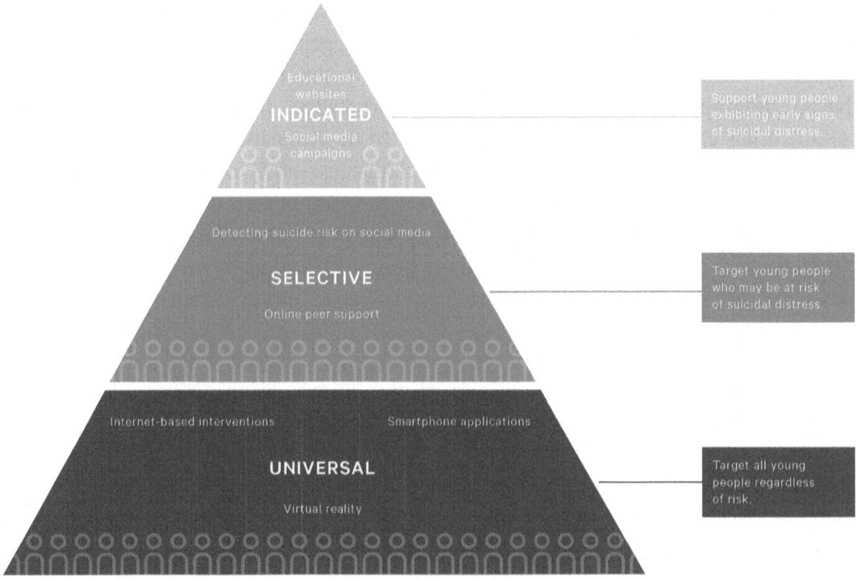

Fig. 8.1 Universal, selective, and indicated interventions using digital technology for youth suicide prevention

interventions may be enhanced by digital technology and the associated ethical and safety issues that must be considered.

8.2 Universal Suicide Prevention Strategies

As noted above, universal interventions target the general population regardless of suicide risk. These interventions typically include restricting access to means or methods of suicide, media guidelines, and programs designed to raise awareness, educate communities, and promote protective factors, including help-seeking. In terms of digital interventions, these may include social media campaigns and the development of educational websites (Rassy et al., 2021).

8.2.1 Social Medial Campaigns

Public health campaigns are among the most widely implemented universal interventions and have been identified as an effective method to disseminate information for suicide prevention (Pirkis et al., 2019). Social media platforms offer an alternative avenue to deliver public health messaging. They can be distributed quickly and reach large numbers of people, particularly those who are geographically dispersed or may be otherwise difficult to engage (Robinson et al., 2016). Online algorithms can be used to optimize the performance of social media campaigns and ensure they reach the target population.

Social media campaigns may be beneficial for targeting young people. Young people are avid social media users and often use these platforms to communicate with their peers and access information, including health-related information (O'Reilly et al., 2019). Evidence from other areas (e.g., mental health stigma and help-seeking) suggests social media campaigns can increase knowledge and awareness and elicit behavior change (Thompson et al., 2021), highlighting the value of delivering messaging where young people spend most of their time (i.e., online).

The evidence base detailing the effectiveness of social media campaigns specifically for suicide prevention is in its infancy. Preliminary evidence suggests social media campaigns (e.g., ManUp social media campaign, Boys Do Cry social media campaign) generate good engagement and increase conversations relating to masculinity and suicide (Schlichthorst et al., 2019; Scotti Requena et al., 2023). However, an increase in suicide tweets in response to social media campaigns (e.g., Bell Let's Talk Day) does not necessarily translate into a decrease in suicide deaths (Côté et al., 2021). #chatsafe, a social media campaign co-designed with young people to encourage safe communication about suicide online, offers promise in this area. A pilot study found #chatsafe to be safe and acceptable and to increase young people's willingness to intervene against suicide online (La Sala et al., 2021). #chatsafe was also tested as a selective intervention targeting young people bereaved by suicide with similar findings (La Sala et al., 2023). A randomised controlled trial of the #chatsafe social media campaign is currently underway and will provide additional insight into the effectiveness of social media campaigns for suicide prevention (Robinson et al., 2023).

8.2.2 Educational Websites

Like social media campaigns, educational websites aim to increase awareness, reduce stigma, and promote help-seeking at a population level. They can be information-based or interactive (Rassy et al., 2021) and often include various features (e.g., personal stories, help-seeking information, links to services). Educational websites are widely available (Tepe & Eker, 2023), but a limited number have been rigorously evaluated. Preliminary evidence suggests educational websites improve suicide prevention-related knowledge (Till et al., 2017) and increase help-seeking (i.e., use of referral links and live chats) (Slay et al., 2021). However, information available on educational websites is not always evidence-based (Lai et al., 2014), and therefore, there is the potential for misinformation to be spread. Ensuring website information is regularly updated and reflects best practices is paramount to prevent the spread of inaccurate information. Creating and promoting educational websites as part of a multi-modal approach may also address this. Given that young people frequently access health information online (O'Reilly et al., 2019), when created and delivered in line with best practices, educational websites offer promise as important tools for youth suicide prevention. However, further research is required to build the evidence base.

Despite the benefits of social media campaigns and educational websites for suicide prevention, safety, and ethical issues must be considered. The potential for social media campaigns to reach large numbers of young people quickly is an important advantage; however, this presents its challenges. Public health practitioners and clinicians cannot monitor how the messaging is received and the subsequent discussion between young people. Given this, it is possible that public health messaging, regardless of the level of care taken to create safe messaging, may elicit unsafe conversations about suicide among young people. Guidelines have been developed to help young people communicate safely online about self-harm and suicide (i.e., the #chatsafe guidelines) (Thorn et al., 2023), and these should be made available to young people during the dissemination of suicide prevention campaigns to address this risk. Importantly, young people can be safely engaged in developing suicide prevention messaging and should be involved in this process (Robinson et al., 2017; Thorn et al., 2020).

8.3 Selective Interventions

Selective interventions are designed to identify and support young people at risk of suicide due to individual (e.g., age, sex, gender identity, presence of mental ill-health, exposure to suicide) or environmental (e.g., job loss, lack of access to health-care, stigma associated with help-seeking) factors (World Health Organization, 2014). Selective interventions using digital technologies are wide-ranging and include detecting suicide risk on social media and online peer support groups.

8.3.1 Detecting Suicide Risk on Social Media

Detecting suicide risk (i.e., screening for suicide risk) has been identified as an important strategy for suicide prevention (World Health Organization, 2021a, b). Screening aims to identify at-risk young people and connect them to appropriate services. Traditionally, detecting suicide risk has occurred within health and education settings (Horowitz, 2021; Scott et al., 2010). However, as noted above, many young people at risk for suicide are not engaged with health services (Walby et al., 2018). Even when young people are engaged, clinicians must administer a risk assessment measure, which they may not have the knowledge or resources to do, and the risk assessment tools must adequately identify risk. Despite the availability of a wide range of risk assessment tools, these tools are not always accurate, rendering the prediction of suicide difficult (Whiting & Fazel, 2019). Furthermore, detecting suicide risks in health and education settings requires young people to disclose their distress or intention to harm (Coppersmith et al., 2018), which they may be reluctant to do.

That said, young people often disclose risk on social media (Marchant et al., 2017; Pourmand et al., 2019), making social media platforms a possible setting to identify suicide risk. Evidence demonstrates that information about individuals' mental health can be derived from the text they generate (Le Glaz et al., 2021). This suggests that text-based screening of social media data may be used to identify young people experiencing suicidal distress. Detecting suicide risk on social media is advantageous as it can be used to identify young people who are not engaged in services, can provide real-time data, and can be used to assess individual and population-level suicide risk (Coppersmith et al., 2018; Woo et al., 2015).

Several studies have demonstrated the value of using Twitter to identify suicide risk. Twitter has been preferred over other social media platforms, given that it is text-based, as opposed to an image-based platform. Machine learning algorithms have been found to accurately differentiate between people who are at suicidal risk and those who are not (Braithwaite et al., 2016). Suicide Artificial Intelligence Prediction Heuristic, an algorithm created from publicly available Twitter data, was found to effectively identify suicide risk up to three weeks prior to an event (Roy et al., 2020). Suicide risk, derived from text-based Twitter data, has also been associated with suicide deaths at the population level (Jashinsky et al., 2014). Twitter-identified suicide risk was associated with suicide death over 10 years (January 2013–December 2022) in Japan (Wang et al., 2023) and geographic-specific suicide rates over 3 months in the United States (O'Dea et al., 2015). There is also evidence to suggest suicide risk can be identified using data from other social media platforms, including Weibo (Cheng et al., 2017), Facebook (Ophir et al., 2020), and Instagram (Lekkas et al., 2021).

Detecting suicide risk using social media data offers promise, given its ability to identify young people who are not engaged with health or social services. However, this approach raises several ethical issues. First and foremost, a clear trade-off between privacy and prevention must be considered (Coppersmith et al., 2018). Detecting suicide risk on social media would require an opt-in process (i.e., individuals actively consent for their data to be used) or an opt-out process (i.e., all data is used unless individuals explicitly ask for their data to be removed). Detecting suicide risk through an opt-out process has greater reach and can capture individuals who are disengaged from other services; however, this comes at a cost to individual privacy.

In contrast, the reach of a system operating in an opt-in process would be significantly reduced and would likely only capture those already engaged in services (Coppersmith et al., 2018). Secondly, if social media is used to detect suicide risk, precise response mechanisms and referral pathways must be in place. Further research is required to determine how social media screening programs could be implemented. It may be worth evaluating systems through an opt-in consent process before deciding if large-scale screening programs would be feasible.

8.3.2 Online Peer Support

Online environments offer an alternative environment for young people at risk of suicide to access peer support. Peer support is a system of giving and receiving help centered around sharing common life experiences and situations (Mead et al., 2001). It is recognized as an important strategy for mental health and suicide prevention (Department of Health and Aged Care, 2020).

Peer support allows young people to connect with their peers, share and seek advice, and provide emotional support (Ali et al., 2015). Peer support is often considered a selective intervention but may be categorized as an indicated intervention when delivered as part of a therapeutic intervention (see discussion below). Peer support offers an alternative to support provided within traditional health services and may delivered across several contexts, including schools, community settings, and online (Schlichthorst et al., 2020). Online peer support is an important tool for young people, given that much of their communication and social interaction occurs online (Gomez-Baya et al., 2019). Online peer support can take several forms, including online forums, chatrooms, video calls, and dedicated online support groups, and offers many benefits, including accessibility and anonymity.

Both formally and informally, online peer support has been widely implemented and is viewed as feasible and acceptable (Abou Seif et al., 2022; Drysdale et al., 2022). Preliminary evidence suggests online peer-to-peer interventions for youth mental health may be effective (Ali et al., 2015; Richard et al., 2022). However, limited studies have been conducted to examine its effectiveness for suicide prevention specifically. One exception is Kooth, a moderated online platform providing access to peer and professional support that has been associated with a reduction in suicidal ideation, self-harm, and psychological distress (Stevens et al., 2022). Participants who only used the community aspects of Kooth (e.g., peer support) had similar outcomes to those who sought professional support through the app.

The challenges of online peer support, particularly on platforms that are not monitored, must be acknowledged. Evidence suggests online peer support groups may lead to pro-suicide groups or may normalize maladaptive coping mechanisms (Boehm, 2015; Stevens et al., 2022). Furthermore, online support groups may be triggering, and hearing the stories of peers may increase the burden and psychological distress (Abou Seif et al., 2022). It is suggested that the presence of an online moderator may mitigate some of these risks (Abou Seif et al., 2022; Boehm, 2015). The #chatsafe guidelines (see above) also include guidance for moderators of online peer support forums (Thorn et al., 2023) and, if accessible on platforms that facilitate online peer support, may mitigate some of these challenges. The online safety of young people requires a comprehensive and collaborative effort, and online platforms, technology companies, and policymakers have a responsibility to ensure regulations are in place to ensure the online environment, including platforms that facilitate peer support, is safe. Despite these challenges, online peer support offers promise as a strategy for suicide prevention, and future research should explore this potential.

8.4 Indicated Interventions

Indicated interventions are targeted approaches that aim to provide more intensive and tailored support to young people already displaying suicide-related thoughts or behaviors (World Health Organization, 2014) and may include a range of strategies (e.g., providing information and therapeutic support, developing and enacting safety plans). Indicated digital technology interventions may include internet-based interventions, smartphone applications, and virtual reality.

8.4.1 Internet-Based Interventions

Internet- or web-based interventions provide information, support, and therapeutic assistance to young people via static and dynamic websites. Many of the available internet-based interventions for youth mental health and suicide are based on traditional (i.e., face-to-face) approaches, including cognitive behavioral therapy (CBT). CBT, when delivered face-to-face, has been found to reduce suicidal thoughts and behaviors (Zalsman et al., 2016) but is not always accessible to young people at heightened risk of suicide.

Internet-based CBT (iCBT) addresses some of the barriers to face-to-face treatment experienced by young people (e.g., stigma-related concerns, accessibility, cost, and geographic isolation). It is often flexible in its delivery (guided or self-guided) and may be implemented within health systems, education settings, and the community at scale (Büscher et al., 2020; Christensen et al., 2014; Leavey & Hawkins, 2017). Guided iCBT involves a clinician or researcher assisting the young person through the program, while self-guided iCBT is initiated and driven by the young person (Christensen et al., 2014).

Evidence suggests that iCBT can be effective in reducing suicidal thoughts. A meta-analysis of six studies found that iCBT interventions explicitly designed to target suicidality were associated with significant reductions in suicidal ideation (Büscher et al., 2020). Subsequent meta-analyses have supported this. Yu et al. (2022) found suicide-specific iCBT to be associated with reductions in suicide ideation across four randomized-controlled trials, including data from 1225 participants. Similarly, Büscher et al. (2022) reported on data from nine randomized-controlled trials finding iCBT to be associated with clinically significant reductions in suicidal ideation. Importantly, effect sizes were comparable to those found for face-to-face CBT, suggesting iCBT may be a suitable alternative to traditional approaches. It is important to note that there is insufficient evidence to comment on the impact of CBT on suicidal behavior (Büscher et al., 2020, 2022; Yu et al., 2022); future research should address this gap. The aforementioned studies (Büscher et al., 2020, 2022; Yu et al., 2022) included two programs designed specifically for young people: LEAP (Hill & Pettit, 2019) and Reframe-IT (Hetrick et al., 2017). The LEAP intervention is a self-guided, internet-based intervention designed to identify perceived burdensomeness as a means of reducing suicidal ideation (Hill & Pettit, 2019). LEAP was designed specifically for adolescents and includes two modules (approximately 30 minutes in duration) delivered approximately one week apart. Reframe-IT is a guided iCBT program administered by school wellbeing staff in the school environment. Reframe-IT contains eight modules delivered over 10 weeks. Reframe-IT has been evaluated in Australian schools (Hetrick et al., 2017) and is currently being trialed across education settings in the United Kingdom (Liverpool John Moores University, 2023) and Chile (Núñez et al., 2022).

Despite the reported benefits of iCBT, the field is in its infancy. The current evidence base has relied on studies with small samples, high attrition, and focused on broader concepts (e.g., depression) rather than suicide specifically. Additional research is required to understand the aspects of iCBT that are conducive to positive outcomes (e.g., guided or self-guided), the optimal duration of interventions (e.g., number and length of modules), sub-groups who benefit most from iCBT and the best settings for delivery (e.g., education settings, health settings, community). Studies indicate poor adherence to web-based interventions (Torok et al., 2020);

therefore, enhancing user engagement is another key issue to address. Co-designing web-based interventions with young people will help ensure that interventions are user-centered and may enhance engagement (Thabrew et al., 2018).

8.4.2 Smartphone Applications

Indicated interventions can also be delivered through smartphone applications (apps). Most adolescents and young adults worldwide have access to a smartphone, making smartphone apps highly accessible tools to deliver indicated interventions (Olff, 2015). These apps can be used in health, education, and community settings to support the delivery of several suicide prevention strategies (Grist et al., 2018; Kennard et al., 2018).

Smartphone apps for suicide prevention are widely available and have been informed by several therapeutic modalities, including acceptance and commitment therapy (Tighe et al., 2017) and dialectical behavior therapy (DBT) (Stallard et al., 2018) and CBT (Bush et al., 2017). As of October 2020, there were 66 mHealth smartphone apps for suicide prevention available on iTunes, Apple Store, and Google Play store (Wilks et al., 2021). Most of these have at least one best practice element (e.g., means safety, support, crisis line access, treatment, safety plan), but none include all five. Evidence has been provided to support the acceptability and feasibility of using smartphone apps (Grist et al., 2018; Thabrew et al., 2023), particularly when they have been co-designed with young people (Hetrick et al., 2018). However, many smartphone apps have not been tested for effectiveness (Sander et al., 2021).

Of the smartphone apps that have been tested, the evidence supporting their effectiveness in reducing suicidal ideation is mixed. BeyondNow, a suicide safety planning app, and LifeBuoy, a self-guided app based on DBT, have been associated with a reduction in suicidal ideation (Melvin et al., 2019; Torok et al., 2022). However, several other smartphone apps have not led to a reduction in suicidal ideation (Bush et al., 2017; Franklin et al., 2016; Kennard et al., 2018; O'Toole et al., 2019; Pauwels et al., 2017; Tighe et al., 2017). These apps provide access to a range of suicide prevention strategies, including psychoeducation, safety planning, and emotional support. Further research is needed to ensure that the potential of smartphone apps is maximized. Studies should be conducted to identify the most effective smartphone app features and the population groups that may receive the most benefit. As with internet-based interventions, maximizing user engagement is paramount.

Embedding digital interventions within clinical services, including internet-based interventions and smartphone apps, presents one opportunity to increase user engagement and enhance their potential benefits. Despite being widely available, digital interventions are rarely embedded within existing services (Cross et al., 2023). Moderated Online Social Therapy (MOST), a digital mental health service for 12- to 25-year-olds, is one exception (Alvarez-Jimenez et al., 2020; Rice et al.,

2018). MOST is embedded in over 80 primary and secondary youth mental health services in Australia (Cross et al., 2023) and is currently being evaluated in the United States, Ireland, and Canada. It is designed to integrate with and enhance existing youth mental health services (Cross et al., 2023) but is not a suicide-specific intervention. MOST provides self-directed therapeutic content, a moderated social networking component, peer workers, and one-on-one support for young people. A rigorous evaluation of MOST is currently underway; however, the social networking component of MOST is safe and free of judgment in a sample of young people who experience suicidal ideation (Bailey et al., 2021).

8.4.3 Virtual Reality

The past decade has seen a rapid advancement of virtual reality (VR) technologies. VR allows users to interact with a computer-generated environment and digital avatars (Bahadur et al., 2023). This typically involves users wearing an enclosed head-mounted device that projects a three-dimensional image (Bell et al., 2020). VR technologies can closely replicate real-world environments, and evidence suggests individuals respond similarly to VR and real-world environments (Bell et al., 2020; Freeman et al., 2017; Rowland et al., 2021). VR environments can be controlled and/or manipulated to monitor stimuli responses in real time and, therefore, may be used for suicide prevention (Bell et al., 2020).

VR has been used in youth mental health to deliver interventions for young people (e.g., treatment-focused VR) and to train clinicians and community members to identify risks and provide support to young people (i.e., assessment-focused VR) (Freeman et al., 2017). A recent systematic review and meta-analysis ($N = 96$ studies) found that simulation-based training for suicide risk assessment improved attitudes, skills, knowledge, and behaviors (Richard et al., 2022). This included but was not limited to VR. Furthermore, clinicians have reported satisfaction with simulation-based training using VR (Bahadur et al., 2023), suggesting that assessment-focused VR may offer an alternative approach to increase clinician confidence and skills in assessing a young person at risk of suicide.

Treatment VR has been used to deliver interventions focusing on several different mental health conditions, including anxiety (Opriş et al., 2012), posttraumatic stress disorder (Kothgassner et al., 2019), and emotional disorders (Rowland et al., 2021). It is most used to deliver exposure therapy and has shown promise. Evidence suggests that VR-delivered interventions may be effective in reducing adverse emotions. A recent systematic review ($N = 20$ studies) reported VR effective in improving stress and negative symptoms; however, this review focused on adult populations (Li Pira et al., 2023).

The application of VR technologies to assess risk and deliver interventions specifically for suicide is relatively new, and the corresponding evidence base is in its infancy. A recent study found that participants experienced a reduction in suicidal ideation after completing a virtual suicide choice task using VR (Caulfield et al.,

2023). The authors concluded that VR might be a safe and feasible platform for assessing suicide behaviors. This study, along with evidence from the field of mental health, suggests that VR offers potential as a tool for suicide prevention. Several projects are currently being conducted to advance the evidence base in this area. Findings from these studies will be paramount in driving the future direction of VR for suicide prevention.

8.5 Challenges of Digital Interventions

Digital platforms allow for streamlining existing prevention and early interventions and creating novel strategies to complement existing approaches. However, these opportunities also present several challenges that must be considered before deciding how to use digital technology for youth suicide prevention.

Social media and other online platforms can disseminate information to large audiences quickly and provide opportunities to facilitate peer support. However, this raises several safety issues. Online environments may propagate misinformation and disinformation, increasing incorrect interpretations of available evidence and decreasing help-seeking (Borges do Nascimento et al., 2022). Individuals and/or groups may distribute information online without following the same ethical and legal standards that healthcare providers must adhere to (Celedonia et al., 2021). Regulations aimed at preventing misinformation and keeping young people safe online vary across geographic locations, and the effectiveness of these regulations depends on enforcement mechanisms and collaboration with industry stakeholders. Suicide prevention professionals and young people highlight the need for collaboration between social media companies and policymakers to reduce the dissemination of harmful content online and to promote safe online environments for young people.

Utilizing digital technologies for suicide prevention also presents issues of privacy and confidentiality. It is paramount that young people feel safe using digital technology and confident that their personal information will remain confidential. For this to happen, stringent data storage and protection processes must exist. Similarly, online platforms or apps may be susceptible to data breaches. Providers must ensure that robust cybersecurity measures exist.

Furthermore, there is a potential for individuals to misuse digital interventions. For example, individuals may impersonate others to gain access to their data or to spread, advertently or inadvertently, pro-suicide information. Secure user authentication processes must be in place to reduce unauthorized access and improve these interventions' overall safety and security.

Barriers to the acceptance, uptake, and use of digital technologies within clinical settings present another key challenge. The ethical and legal issues discussed above may prevent the adoption of indicated digital interventions within clinical settings. Clinician's lack of knowledge and experience in delivering digital interventions presents another important challenge (Feijt et al., 2018). This issue is exacerbated by the limited number of structured clinician training programs (Mendes-Santos et al., 2022). Organizational resources, including limited technical support and prohibitive startup costs, present additional barriers (Graham et al., 2020). The development of structured implementation strategies, often lacking (Graham et al., 2020), is required to combat some of these challenges. Best-practice guidelines for integrating digital tools for young people into clinical care have been recently developed (Bailey et al., 2023), and these should be used to aid the implementation of digital strategies into clinical services.

Digital technology is ever-evolving, and the evidence base cannot keep up with the rapid developments in this area. Ethical issues of studies evaluating digital technologies for suicide prevention (e.g., concerns about potential harm, risk management, recruitment difficulties, conflicting views of ethics committees and researchers, and the impact of inclusion and exclusion criteria for generalizability) create additional barriers (Bailey et al., 2020). As a result, many currently available digital interventions do not have sufficient evidence to support their use as standalone services (Braciszewski, 2021). The current approaches to evaluating digital interventions are time-consuming, highlighting the need for a paradigm shift. More must be done to adapt what is learned from other industries (e.g., technology and software development industry) to ensure the timely and comprehensive evaluation of digital strategies.

8.6 Future Directions

Digital technology has the potential to change the landscape of youth suicide prevention. However, additional research and streamlined evaluation processes are required to realize this potential. The evidence base remains limited in comparison to the rapid pace of technological innovation, with a marked shortage of high-quality studies specifically addressing youth populations (Bell et al., 2020; Freeman et al., 2017). Several other methodological issues are present among the studies that do exist (Melia et al., 2020). There is no standardized measurement of suicide outcomes used across studies, making comparisons difficult (Melia et al., 2020). There is also a tendency to exclude potential participants due to elevated suicide risk, which is guided by safety considerations but may bias outcomes. Future research must address these limitations. Digital interventions should follow Safety by Design principles (eSafety Commissioner, 2023). These principles ensure that user safety and rights are central to designing and developing digital interventions and services. It is also paramount that interventions are co-designed and evaluated with young people, and implementation strategies, as discussed above, are considered from the outset to enhance user engagement and maximize the potential of digital interventions. Guidelines for involving young people with lived experience of suicide in research have been developed and should be utilized by researchers and public health practitioners in this area (Webb et al., 2024).

In summary, many digital strategies for youth suicide prevention address the barriers to traditional suicide prevention approaches and are advantageous in their accessibility, acceptability, and feasibility. Digital interventions have the potential to enhance youth suicide prevention efforts, but these strategies should complement rather than replace existing approaches. Many available interventions have not been rigorously evaluated, and ethical and safety issues frequently arise with new and existing technology. As such, clinicians, public health practitioners, and policymakers should exercise caution when deciding how to integrate digital technology into practice. The decision to implement digital strategies should be evidence-informed and guided by ethical principles.

Acknowledgments DN received funding from ANID—Millennium Science Initiative Program NCS2021_081 and ANID—Fondecy Project N° 1210093.

References

Abou Seif, N., John-Baptiste Bastien, R., Wang, B., Davies, J., Isaken, M., Ball, E., Pitman, A., & Rowe, S. (2022). Effectiveness, acceptability and potential harms of peer support for self-harm in non-clinical settings: Systematic review. *BJPsych Open, 8*(1), e28. https://doi.org/10.1192/bjo.2021.1081

Ali, K., Farrer, L., Gulliver, A., & Griffiths, K. M. (2015). Online peer-to-peer support for young people with mental health problems: A systematic review. *JMIR Mental Health, 2*(2), e19. https://doi.org/10.2196/mental.4418

Alvarez-Jimenez, M., Rice, S., D'Alfonso, S., Leicester, S., Bendall, S., Pryor, I., Russon, P., McEnery, C., Santesteban-Echarri, O., Da Costa, G., Gilbertson, T., Valentine, L., Solves, L., Ratheesh, A., McGorry, P. D., & Gleeson, J. (2020). A novel multimodal digital service (moderated online social therapy+) for help-seeking young people experiencing mental ill-health: Pilot evaluation within a national youth e-mental health service. *Journal of Medical Internet Research, 22*(8), e17155. https://doi.org/10.2196/17155

Anderson, J. K., Howarth, E., Vainre, M., Jones, P. B., & Humphrey, A. (2017). A scoping literature review of service-level barriers for access and engagement with mental health services for children and young people. *Children and Youth Services Review, 77*, 164–176. https://doi.org/10.1016/j.childyouth.2017.04.017

Australian Institute of Health and Welfare. (2023). *Suicide and self-harm monitoring data.*

Bahadur, A. G., Hargreaves, F., Antinucci, R., Sockalingam, S., & Abdool, P. S. (2023). Virtual reality simulation for suicide risk assessment training: Prevalence of adverse effects. *Academic Psychiatry*. https://doi.org/10.1007/s40596-023-01799-1

Bailey, E., Bellairs-Walsh, I., Reavley, N., Gooding, P., Hetrick, S., Rice, S., Boland, A., & Robinson, J. (2023). *Guidelines for integrating digital tools into clinical care for young people at risk of suicide.* https://www.orygen.org.au/Training/Resources/Self-harm-and-suicide-prevention/Guidelines/integrating-digital-tools-into-clinical-care

Bailey, E., Mühlmann, C., Rice, S., Nedeljkovic, M., Alvarez-Jimenez, M., Sander, L., Calear, A. L., Batterham, P. J., & Robinson, J. (2020). Ethical issues and practical barriers in internet-based suicide prevention research: A review and investigator survey. *BMC Medical Ethics, 21*(1), 37. https://doi.org/10.1186/s12910-020-00479-1

Bailey, E., Robinson, J., Alvarez-Jimenez, M., Nedeljkovic, M., Valentine, L., Bendall, S., D'Alfonso, S., Gilbertson, T., McKechnie, B., & Rice, S. (2021). Moderated online social therapy for young people with active suicidal ideation: Qualitative study. *Journal of Medical Internet Research, 23*(4), e24260. https://doi.org/10.2196/24260

Bell, I. H., Nicholas, J., Alvarez-Jimenez, M., Thompson, A., & Valmaggia, L. (2020). Virtual reality as a clinical tool in mental health research and practice. *Dialogues in Clinical Neuroscience, 22*(2), 169–177. https://doi.org/10.31887/DCNS.2020.22.2/lvalmaggia

Boehm, N. (2015). *Responding to suicidal ideations in online peer support groups*. Colorado State University.

Borges do Nascimento, I. J., Beatriz Pizarro, A., Almeida, J., Azzopardi-Muscat, N., André Gonçalves, M., Björklund, M., & Novillo-Ortiz, D. (2022). Infodemics and health misinformation: A systematic review of reviews. *Bulletin of the World Health Organization, 100*(9), 544–561. https://doi.org/10.2471/BLT.21.287654

Braciszewski, J. M. (2021). Digital technology for suicide prevention. *Advances in Psychiatry and Behavioral Health, 1*(1), 53–65. https://doi.org/10.1016/j.ypsc.2021.05.008

Braithwaite, S. R., Giraud-Carrier, C., West, J., Barnes, M. D., & Hanson, C. L. (2016). Validating machine learning algorithms for twitter data against established measures of suicidality. *JMIR Mental Health, 3*(2), e21. https://doi.org/10.2196/mental.4822

Brown, A., Rice, S. M., Rickwood, D. J., & Parker, A. G. (2016). Systematic review of barriers and facilitators to accessing and engaging with mental health care among at-risk young people. *Asia-Pacific Psychiatry, 8*(1), 3–22. https://doi.org/10.1111/appy.12199

Büscher, R., Beisemann, M., Doebler, P., Micklitz, H. M., Kerkhof, A., Cuijpers, P., Batterham, P. J., Calear, A. L., Christensen, H., De Jaegere, E., Domhardt, M., Erlangsen, A., Eylem van Bergeijk, O., Hill, R., Lungu, A., Mühlmann, C., Pettit, J. W., Portzky, G., Steubl, L. S., et al. (2022). Digital cognitive–behavioural therapy to reduce suicidal ideation and behaviours: A systematic review and meta-analysis of individual participant data. *Evidence Based Mental Health, 25*(e1), e8–e17. https://doi.org/10.1136/ebmental-2022-300540

Büscher, R., Torok, M., Terhorst, Y., & Sander, L. (2020). Internet-based cognitive behavioral therapy to reduce suicidal ideation. *JAMA Network Open, 3*(4), e203933. https://doi.org/10.1001/jamanetworkopen.2020.3933

Bush, N. E., Smolenski, D. J., Denneson, L. M., Williams, H. B., Thomas, E. K., & Dobscha, S. K. (2017). A virtual hope box: Randomized controlled trial of a smartphone app for emotional regulation and coping with distress. *Psychiatric Services, 68*(4), 330–336. https://doi.org/10.1176/appi.ps.201600283

Caulfield, N. M., Bauer, B. W., Fergerson, A., Karnick, A. T., & Capron, D. W. (2023). *Examining the safety and feasibility of using virtual reality to assess suicide risk* (Preprint). https://assets-eu.researchsquare.com/files/rs-3219176/v1/2261cf06-97be-4668-9f2c-669866bafb16.pdf?c=1696395149

Celedonia, K. L., Corrales Compagnucci, M., Minssen, T., & Lowery Wilson, M. (2021). Legal, ethical, and wider implications of suicide risk detection systems in social media platforms. *Journal of Law and the Biosciences, 8*(1). https://doi.org/10.1093/jlb/lsab021

Cheng, Q., Li, T. M., Kwok, C.-L., Zhu, T., & Yip, P. S. (2017). Assessing suicide risk and emotional distress in Chinese social media: A text mining and machine learning study. *Journal of Medical Internet Research, 19*(7), e243. https://doi.org/10.2196/jmir.7276

Christensen, H., Batterham, P., & O'Dea, B. (2014). E-Health interventions for suicide prevention. *International Journal of Environmental Research and Public Health, 11*(8), 8193–8212. https://doi.org/10.3390/ijerph110808193

Coppersmith, G., Leary, R., Crutchley, P., & Fine, A. (2018). Natural language processing of social media as screening for suicide risk. In *Biomedical informatics insights* (Vol. 10, p. 1178222618792860). SAGE. https://doi.org/10.1177/1178222618792860

Côté, D., Williams, M., Zaheer, R., Niederkrotenthaler, T., Schaffer, A., & Sinyor, M. (2021). Suicide-related Twitter content in response to a national mental health awareness campaign and the association between the campaign and suicide rates in Ontario. *The Canadian Journal of Psychiatry, 66*(5), 460–467. https://doi.org/10.1177/0706743720982428

Cross, S. P., Nicholas, J., Bell, I. H., Mangelsdorf, S., Valentine, L., Thompson, A., Gleeson, J. F., & Alvarez-Jimenez, M. (2023). Integrating digital interventions with clinical practice in youth mental health services. *Australasian Psychiatry, 31*(3), 302–305. https://doi.org/10.1177/10398562231169365

Department of Health and Aged Care. (2020). *National suicide prevention strategy for Australia's health system* (2020–2023). https://www.health.gov.au/resources/publications/national-suicide-prevention-strategy-for-australias-health-system-2020-2023?language=en

Drysdale, M. T. B., McBeath, M. L., & Callaghan, S. A. (2022). The feasibility and impact of online peer support on the well-being of higher education students. *The Journal of Mental Health Training, Education and Practice, 17*(3), 206–217. https://doi.org/10.1108/JMHTEP-02-2021-0012

eSafety Commissioner. (2023). *Safety by design*. https://www.esafety.gov.au/industry/safety-by-design

Feijt, M. A., de Kort, Y. A., Bongers, I. M., & IJsselsteijn, W. A. (2018). Perceived drivers and barriers to the adoption of eMental Health by psychologists: The construction of the levels of adoption of eMental Health Model. *Journal of Medical Internet Research, 20*(4), e153. https://doi.org/10.2196/jmir.9485

Franklin, J. C., Fox, K. R., Franklin, C. R., Kleiman, E. M., Ribeiro, J. D., Jaroszewski, A. C., Hooley, J. M., & Nock, M. K. (2016). A brief mobile app reduces nonsuicidal and suicidal self-injury: Evidence from three randomized controlled trials. *Journal of Consulting and Clinical Psychology, 84*(6), 544–557. https://doi.org/10.1037/ccp0000093

Freeman, D., Reeve, S., Robinson, A., Ehlers, A., Clark, D., Spanlang, B., & Slater, M. (2017). Virtual reality in the assessment, understanding, and treatment of mental health disorders. *Psychological Medicine, 47*(14), 2393–2400. https://doi.org/10.1017/S003329171700040X

Gomez-Baya, D., Rubio-Gonzalez, A., & Gaspar de Matos, M. (2019). Online communication, peer relationships and school victimisation: A one-year longitudinal study during middle adolescence. *International Journal of Adolescence and Youth, 24*(2), 199–211. https://doi.org/10.1080/02673843.2018.1509793

Graham, A. K., Lattie, E. G., Powell, B. J., Lyon, A. R., Smith, J. D., Schueller, S. M., Stadnick, N. A., Brown, C. H., & Mohr, D. C. (2020). Implementation strategies for digital mental health interventions in health care settings. *American Psychologist, 75*(8), 1080–1092. https://doi.org/10.1037/amp0000686

Grist, R., Porter, J., & Stallard, P. (2018). Acceptability, use, and safety of a Mobile Phone App (BlueIce) for young people who self-harm: Qualitative study of service users' experience. *JMIR Mental Health, 5*(1), e16. https://doi.org/10.2196/mental.8779

Hetrick, S. E., Robinson, J., Burge, E., Blandon, R., Mobilio, B., Rice, S. M., Simmons, M. B., Alvarez-Jimenez, M., Goodrich, S., & Davey, C. G. (2018). Youth codesign of a mobile phone app to facilitate self-monitoring and management of mood symptoms in young people with major depression, suicidal ideation, and self-harm. *JMIR Mental Health, 5*(1), e9. https://doi.org/10.2196/mental.9041

Hetrick, S. E., Yuen, H. P., Bailey, E., Cox, G. R., Templer, K., Rice, S. M., Bendall, S., & Robinson, J. (2017). Internet-based cognitive behavioural therapy for young people with suicide-related behaviour (Reframe-IT): A randomised controlled trial. *Evidence Based Mental Health, 20*(3), 76–82. https://doi.org/10.1136/eb-2017-102719

Hill, R. M., & Pettit, J. W. (2019). Pilot randomized controlled trial of LEAP: A selective preventive intervention to reduce adolescents' perceived burdensomeness. *Journal of Clinical Child & Adolescent Psychology, 48*(sup1), S45–S56. https://doi.org/10.1080/15374416.2016.1188705

Horowitz, L. (2021). Screening for suicide risk in medical settings: From research to implementation. *European Psychiatry, 64*(S1), S178–S179. https://doi.org/10.1192/j.eurpsy.2021.473

Jashinsky, J., Burton, S. H., Hanson, C. L., West, J., Giraud-Carrier, C., Barnes, M. D., & Argyle, T. (2014). Tracking suicide risk factors through Twitter in the US. *Crisis, 35*(1), 51–59. https://doi.org/10.1027/0227-5910/a000234

Kennard, B. D., Goldstein, T., Foxwell, A. A., McMakin, D. L., Wolfe, K., Biernesser, C., Moorehead, A., Douaihy, A., Zullo, L., Wentroble, E., Owen, V., Zelazny, J., Iyengar, S., Porta,

G., & Brent, D. (2018). As Safe as Possible (ASAP): A brief app-supported inpatient intervention to prevent postdischarge suicidal behavior in hospitalized suicidal adolescents. *American Journal of Psychiatry, 175*(9), 864–872. https://doi.org/10.1176/appi.ajp.2018.17101151

Kothgassner, O. D., Goreis, A., Kafka, J. X., Van Eickels, R. L., Plener, P. L., & Felnhofer, A. (2019). Virtual reality exposure therapy for posttraumatic stress disorder (PTSD): A meta-analysis. *European Journal of Psychotraumatology, 10*(1). https://doi.org/10.1080/20008198.2019.1654782

La Sala, L., Pirkis, J., Cooper, C., Hill, N. T. M., Lamblin, M., Rajaram, G., Rice, S., Teh, Z., Thorn, P., Zahan, R., & Robinson, J. (2023). Acceptability and potential impact of the #chatsafe suicide postvention response among young people who have been exposed to suicide: Pilot study. *JMIR Human Factors, 10*, e44535. https://doi.org/10.2196/44535

La Sala, L., Teh, Z., Lamblin, M., Rajaram, G., Rice, S., Hill, N. T. M., Thorn, P., Krysinska, K., & Robinson, J. (2021). Can a social media intervention improve online communication about suicide? A feasibility study examining the acceptability and potential impact of the #chatsafe campaign. *PLoS One, 16*(6), e0253278. https://doi.org/10.1371/journal.pone.0253278

Lai, M. H., Maniam, T., Chan, L. F., & Ravindran, A. V. (2014). Caught in the web: A review of web-based suicide prevention. *Journal of Medical Internet Research, 16*(1), e30. https://doi.org/10.2196/jmir.2973

Le Glaz, A., Haralambous, Y., Kim-Dufor, D.-H., Lenca, P., Billot, R., Ryan, T. C., Marsh, J., DeVylder, J., Walter, M., Berrouiguet, S., & Lemey, C. (2021). Machine learning and natural language processing in Mental Health: Systematic review. *Journal of Medical Internet Research, 23*(5), e15708. https://doi.org/10.2196/15708

Leavey, K., & Hawkins, R. (2017). Is cognitive behavioural therapy effective in reducing suicidal ideation and behaviour when delivered face-to-face or via e-health? A systematic review and meta-analysis. *Cognitive Behaviour Therapy, 46*(5), 353–374. https://doi.org/10.1080/16506073.2017.1332095

Lekkas, D., Klein, R. J., & Jacobson, N. C. (2021). Predicting acute suicidal ideation on Instagram using ensemble machine learning models. *Internet Interventions, 25*, 100424. https://doi.org/10.1016/j.invent.2021.100424

Li Pira, G., Aquilini, B., Davoli, A., Grandi, S., & Ruini, C. (2023). The use of virtual reality interventions to promote positive mental health: Systematic literature review. *JMIR Mental Health, 10*, e44998. https://doi.org/10.2196/44998

Liverpool John Moores University. (2023). *Multi-Modal Approach to Preventing Suicide in Schools* (MAPSS). https://www.ljmu.ac.uk/research/centres-and-institutes/institute-of-health-research/expertise/suicide-and-self-harm/multi-modal-approach-to-preventing-suicide-in-schools

Luxton, D. D., June, J. D., & Kinn, J. T. (2011). Technology-based suicide prevention: Current applications and future directions. *Telemedicine and e-Health, 17*(1), 50–54. https://doi.org/10.1089/tmj.2010.0091

Marchant, A., Hawton, K., Stewart, A., Montgomery, P., Singaravelu, V., Lloyd, K., Purdy, N., Daine, K., & John, A. (2017). A systematic review of the relationship between internet use, self-harm and suicidal behaviour in young people: The good, the bad and the unknown. *PLoS One, 12*(8), e0181722. https://doi.org/10.1371/journal.pone.0181722

Mead, S., Hilton, D., & Curtis, L. (2001). Peer support: A theoretical perspective. *Psychiatric Rehabilitation Journal, 25*(2), 134–141. https://doi.org/10.1037/h0095032

Melia, R., Francis, K., Hickey, E., Bogue, J., Duggan, J., O'Sullivan, M., & Young, K. (2020). Mobile health technology interventions for suicide prevention: Systematic review. *JMIR mHealth and uHealth, 8*(1), e12516. https://doi.org/10.2196/12516

Melvin, G. A., Gresham, D., Beaton, S., Coles, J., Tonge, B. J., Gordon, M. S., & Stanley, B. (2019). Evaluating the feasibility and effectiveness of an Australian Safety Planning Smartphone Application: A pilot study within a tertiary mental health service. *Suicide and Life-threatening Behavior, 49*(3), 846–858. https://doi.org/10.1111/sltb.12490

Mendes-Santos, C., Nunes, F., Weiderpass, E., Santana, R., & Andersson, G. (2022). Understanding mental health professionals' perspectives and practices regarding the implementation of

digital mental health: qualitative study. *JMIR Formative Research, 6*(4), e32558. https://doi.org/10.2196/32558
Núñez, D., Gaete, J., Meza, D., Andaur, J., & Robinson, J. (2022). Testing the effectiveness of a blended intervention to reduce suicidal ideation among school adolescents in Chile: A protocol for a cluster randomized controlled trial. *International Journal of Environmental Research and Public Health, 19*(7), 3947. https://doi.org/10.3390/ijerph19073947
O'Dea, B., Wan, S., Batterham, P. J., Calear, A. L., Paris, C., & Christensen, H. (2015). Detecting suicidality on Twitter. *Internet Interventions, 2*(2), 183–188. https://doi.org/10.1016/j.invent.2015.03.005
O'Reilly, M., Dogra, N., Hughes, J., Reilly, P., George, R., & Whiteman, N. (2019). Potential of social media in promoting mental health in adolescents. *Health Promotion International, 34*(5), 981–991. https://doi.org/10.1093/heapro/day056
O'Toole, M. S., Arendt, M. B., & Pedersen, C. M. (2019). Testing an App-assisted treatment for suicide prevention in a randomized controlled trial: Effects on suicide risk and depression. *Behavior Therapy, 50*(2), 421–429. https://doi.org/10.1016/j.beth.2018.07.007
Olff, M. (2015). Mobile mental health: A challenging research agenda. *European Journal of Psychotraumatology, 6*(1). https://doi.org/10.3402/ejpt.v6.27882
Ophir, Y., Tikochinski, R., Asterhan, C. S. C., Sisso, I., & Reichart, R. (2020). Deep neural networks detect suicide risk from textual facebook posts. *Scientific Reports, 10*(1), 16685. https://doi.org/10.1038/s41598-020-73917-0
Opriş, D., Pintea, S., García-Palacios, A., Botella, C., Szamosközi, Ş., & David, D. (2012). Virtual reality exposure therapy in anxiety disorders: A quantitative meta-analysis. *Depression and Anxiety, 29*(2), 85–93. https://doi.org/10.1002/da.20910
Osborne, D., De Boer, K., Meyer, D., & Nedeljkovic, M. (2023). Raising suicide in medical appointments—Barriers and facilitators experienced by young adults and GPs: A mixed-methods systematic review. *International Journal of Environmental Research and Public Health, 20*(1), 822. https://doi.org/10.3390/ijerph20010822
Pauwels, K., Aerts, S., Muijzers, E., De Jaegere, E., van Heeringen, K., & Portzky, G. (2017). BackUp: Development and evaluation of a smart-phone application for coping with suicidal crises. *PLoS One, 12*(6), e0178144. https://doi.org/10.1371/journal.pone.0178144
Pirkis, J., Rossetto, A., Nicholas, A., Ftanou, M., Robinson, J., & Reavley, N. (2019). Suicide prevention media campaigns: A systematic literature review. *Health Communication, 34*(4), 402–414. https://doi.org/10.1080/10410236.2017.1405484
Pourmand, A., Roberson, J., Caggiula, A., Monsalve, N., Rahimi, M., & Torres-Llenza, V. (2019). Social media and suicide: A review of technology-based epidemiology and risk assessment. *Telemedicine and e-Health, 25*(10), 880–888. https://doi.org/10.1089/tmj.2018.0203
Radez, J., Reardon, T., Creswell, C., Lawrence, P. J., Evdoka-Burton, G., & Waite, P. (2021). Why do children and adolescents (not) seek and access professional help for their mental health problems? A systematic review of quantitative and qualitative studies. *European Child & Adolescent Psychiatry, 30*(2), 183–211. https://doi.org/10.1007/s00787-019-01469-4
Rassy, J., Bardon, C., Dargis, L., Côté, L.-P., Corthésy-Blondin, L., Mörch, C.-M., & Labelle, R. (2021). Information and communication technology use in suicide prevention: Scoping review. *Journal of Medical Internet Research, 23*(5), e25288. https://doi.org/10.2196/25288
Rice, S., Gleeson, J., Leicester, S., Bendall, S., D'Alfonso, S., Gilbertson, T., Killackey, E., Parker, A., Lederman, R., Wadley, G., Santesteban-Echarri, O., Pryor, I., Mawren, D., Ratheesh, A., & Alvarez-Jimenez, M. (2018). Implementation of the Enhanced Moderated Online Social Therapy (MOST+) model within a national youth e-mental health service (eheadspace): Protocol for a single group pilot study for help-seeking young people. *JMIR Research Protocols, 7*(2), e48. https://doi.org/10.2196/resprot.8813
Richard, J., Rebinsky, R., Suresh, R., Kubic, S., Carter, A., Cunningham, J. E. A., Ker, A., Williams, K., & Sorin, M. (2022). Scoping review to evaluate the effects of peer support on the mental health of young adults. *BMJ Open, 12*(8), e061336. https://doi.org/10.1136/bmjopen-2022-061336

Robinson, J., Bailey, E., Hetrick, S., Paix, S., O'Donnell, M., Cox, G., Ftanou, M., & Skehan, J. (2017). Developing social media-based suicide prevention messages in partnership with young people: Exploratory study. *JMIR Mental Health, 4*(4), e40. https://doi.org/10.2196/mental.7847

Robinson, J., Cox, G., Bailey, E., Hetrick, S., Rodrigues, M., Fisher, S., & Herrman, H. (2016). Social media and suicide prevention: A systematic review. *Early Intervention in Psychiatry, 10*(2), 103–121. https://doi.org/10.1111/eip.12229

Robinson, J., La Sala, L., Cooper, C., Spittal, M., Rice, S., Lamblin, M., Brown, E., Nolan, H., Battersby-Coulter, R., Rajaram, G., Thorn, P., Pirkis, J., May-Finlay, S., Silenzio, V., Skehan, J., Krysinska, K., & Bellairs-Walsh, I. (2023). Testing the impact of the #chatsafe intervention on young people's ability to communicate safely about suicide on social media: Protocol for a randomized controlled trial. *JMIR Research Protocols, 12*, e44300. https://doi.org/10.2196/44300

Rowland, D. P., Casey, L. M., Ganapathy, A., Cassimatis, M., & Clough, B. A. (2021). A decade in review: A systematic review of virtual reality interventions for emotional disorders. *Psychosocial Intervention, 31*(1), 1–20. https://doi.org/10.5093/pi2021a8

Roy, A., Nikolitch, K., McGinn, R., Jinah, S., Klement, W., & Kaminsky, Z. A. (2020). A machine learning approach predicts future risk to suicidal ideation from social media data. *npj Digital Medicine, 3*(1), 78. https://doi.org/10.1038/s41746-020-0287-6

Ruch, D. A., Sheftall, A. H., Schlagbaum, P., Rausch, J., Campo, J. V., & Bridge, J. A. (2019). Trends in suicide among youth aged 10 to 19 years in the United States, 1975 to 2016. *JAMA Network Open, 2*(5), e193886. https://doi.org/10.1001/jamanetworkopen.2019.3886

Sander, L. B., Lemor, M.-L., Van der Sloot, R. J. A., De Jaegere, E., Büscher, R., Messner, E.-M., Baumeister, H., & Terhorst, Y. (2021). A systematic evaluation of mobile health applications for the prevention of suicidal behavior or non-suicidal self-injury. *Frontiers in Digital Health, 3*. https://doi.org/10.3389/fdgth.2021.689692

Schlichthorst, M., King, K., Reifels, L., Phelps, A., & Pirkis, J. (2019). Using social media networks to engage men in conversations on masculinity and suicide: Content analysis of man up Facebook Campaign Data. *Social Media + Society, 5*(4), 205630511988001. https://doi.org/10.1177/2056305119880019

Schlichthorst, M., Ozols, I., Reifels, L., & Morgan, A. (2020). Lived experience peer support programs for suicide prevention: A systematic scoping review. *International Journal of Mental Health Systems, 14*(1), 65. https://doi.org/10.1186/s13033-020-00396-1

Scott, M., Wilcox, H., Huo, Y., Turner, J. B., Fisher, P., & Shaffer, D. (2010). School-based screening for suicide risk: Balancing costs and benefits. *American Journal of Public Health, 100*(9), 1648–1652. https://doi.org/10.2105/AJPH.2009.175224

Scotti Requena, S., Pirkis, J., Currier, D., Conway, M., Lee, S., Turnure, J., Cummins, J., & Nicholas, A. (2023). An evaluation of the boys do cry suicide prevention media campaign on Twitter: Mixed methods approach. *JMIR Formative Research, 7*, e49325. https://doi.org/10.2196/49325

Selkie, E., Adkins, V., Masters, E., Bajpai, A., & Shumer, D. (2020). Transgender adolescents' uses of social media for social support. *Journal of Adolescent Health, 66*(3), 275–280. https://doi.org/10.1016/j.jadohealth.2019.08.011

Slay, P. D., Castille, K. W., Hong, E., Polizzi, N., & Hoyt, T. (2021). Enhancing suicide prevention outreach via mobile-enabled website design. *Suicide and Life-threatening Behavior, 51*(2), 229–236. https://doi.org/10.1111/sltb.12698

Stallard, P., Porter, J., & Grist, R. (2018). A Smartphone App (BlueIce) for young people who self-harm: Open phase 1 pre-post trial. *JMIR mHealth and uHealth, 6*(1), e32. https://doi.org/10.2196/mhealth.8917

Stevens, M., Cartagena Farías, J., Mindel, C., D'Amico, F., & Evans-Lacko, S. (2022). Pilot evaluation to assess the effectiveness of youth peer community support via the Kooth online mental wellbeing website. *BMC Public Health, 22*(1), 1903. https://doi.org/10.1186/s12889-022-14223-4

Tepe, Ç. Ş., & Eker, F. (2023). Content analysis of suicide prevention web pages from perspective of preventive psychiatric approaches. *Current Psychology*. https://doi.org/10.1007/s12144-023-04496-2

Thabrew, H., Fleming, T., Hetrick, S., & Merry, S. (2018). Co-design of eHealth interventions with children and young people. *Frontiers in Psychiatry, 9*. https://doi.org/10.3389/fpsyt.2018.00481

Thabrew, H., Kumar, H., & Steadman, E. (2023). Acceptability and feasibility of "village," a digital communication app for young people experiencing low mood, thoughts of self-harm, and suicidal ideation to obtain support from family and friends: Mixed methods pilot open trial. *JMIR Formative Research, 7*, e41273. https://doi.org/10.2196/41273

Thompson, A., Hollis, S., Herman, K. C., Reinke, W. M., Hawley, K., & Magee, S. (2021). Evaluation of a social media campaign on youth mental health stigma and help-seeking. *School Psychology Review, 50*(1), 36–41. https://doi.org/10.1080/2372966X.2020.1838873

Thorn, P., Hill, N. T., Lamblin, M., Teh, Z., Battersby-Coulter, R., Rice, S., Bendall, S., Gibson, K. L., Finlay, S. M., Blandon, R., de Souza, L., West, A., Cooksey, A., Sciglitano, J., Goodrich, S., & Robinson, J. (2020). Developing a suicide prevention social media campaign with young people (The #Chatsafe Project): Co-design approach. *JMIR Mental Health, 7*(5), e17520. https://doi.org/10.2196/17520

Thorn, P., McKay, S., Hemming, L., Reavley, N., La Sala, L., Sabo, A., McCormack, T., Battersby-Coulter, R., Cooper, C., & Lamblin, M. (2023). *#chatsafe: A young person's guide to communicating safely online about self-harm and suicide*: Edition two. https://www.orygen.org.au/chatsafe

Tighe, J., Shand, F., Ridani, R., Mackinnon, A., De La Mata, N., & Christensen, H. (2017). Ibobbly mobile health intervention for suicide prevention in Australian Indigenous youth: A pilot randomised controlled trial. *BMJ Open, 7*(1), e013518. https://doi.org/10.1136/bmjopen-2016-013518

Till, B., Tran, U. S., Voracek, M., & Niederkrotenthaler, T. (2017). Beneficial and harmful effects of educative suicide prevention websites: Randomised controlled trial exploring Papageno vs Werther effects. *British Journal of Psychiatry, 211*(2), 109–115. https://doi.org/10.1192/bjp.bp.115.177394

Torok, M., Han, J., Baker, S., Werner-Seidler, A., Wong, I., Larsen, M. E., & Christensen, H. (2020). Suicide prevention using self-guided digital interventions: A systematic review and meta-analysis of randomised controlled trials. *The Lancet Digital Health, 2*(1), e25–e36. https://doi.org/10.1016/S2589-7500(19)30199-2

Torok, M., Han, J., McGillivray, L., Wong, Q., Werner-Seidler, A., O'Dea, B., Calear, A., & Christensen, H. (2022). The effect of a therapeutic smartphone application on suicidal ideation in young adults: Findings from a randomized controlled trial in Australia. *PLoS Medicine, 19*(5), e1003978. https://doi.org/10.1371/journal.pmed.1003978

Walby, F. A., Myhre, M. Ø., & Kildahl, A. T. (2018). Contact with mental health services prior to suicide: A systematic review and meta-analysis. *Psychiatric Services, 69*(7), 751–759. https://doi.org/10.1176/appi.ps.201700475

Wang, S., Ning, H., Huang, X., Xiao, Y., Zhang, M., Yang, E. F., Sadahiro, Y., Liu, Y., Li, Z., Hu, T., Fu, X., Li, Z., & Zeng, Y. (2023). Public surveillance of social media for suicide using advanced deep learning models in Japan: Time series study from 2012 to 2022. *Journal of Medical Internet Research, 25*, e47225. https://doi.org/10.2196/47225

Webb, M., Cooper, C., Hemming, L., Dalton, A., Unity, E., Simmons, M. B., Bendall, S., & Robinson, J. (2024). Involving young people with lived and living experience of suicide in suicide research. *Crisis, 45*(4), 263–270. https://doi.org/10.1027/0227-5910/a000938

Whiting, D., & Fazel, S. (2019). How accurate are suicide risk prediction models? Asking the right questions for clinical practice. *Evidence Based Mental Health, 22*(3), 125–128. https://doi.org/10.1136/ebmental-2019-300102

Wilks, C. R., Chu, C., Sim, D., Lovell, J., Gutierrez, P., Joiner, T., Kessler, R. C., & Nock, M. K. (2021). User engagement and usability of suicide prevention apps: Systematic search in app stores and content analysis. *JMIR Formative Research, 5*(7), e27018. https://doi.org/10.2196/27018

Woo, H., Cho, Y., Shim, E., Lee, K., & Song, G. (2015). Public Trauma after the Sewol Ferry Disaster: The role of social media in understanding the public mood. *International Journal of Environmental Research and Public Health, 12*(9), 10974–10983. https://doi.org/10.3390/ijerph120910974

World Health Organization. (2014). *Preventing suicide: A global imperative.* https://www.who.int/publications/i/item/9789241564779

World Health Organization. (2021a). *LIVE LIFE: An implementation guide for suicide prevention in countries.* World Health Organization.

World Health Organization. (2021b). *Suicide worldwide in 2019: Global health estimates.* https://www.who.int/publications/i/item/9789240026643.

Yu, T., Hu, D., Teng, F., Mao, J., Xu, K., Han, Y., Liu, Y., & Wu, M. (2022). Effectiveness of internet-based cognitive behavioral therapy for suicide: A systematic review and meta-analysis of RCTs. *Psychology, Health & Medicine, 27*(10), 2186–2203. https://doi.org/10.1080/13548506.2021.1930073

Zalsman, G., Hawton, K., Wasserman, D., van Heeringen, K., Arensman, E., Sarchiapone, M., Carli, V., Höschl, C., Barzilay, R., Balazs, J., Purebl, G., Kahn, J. P., Sáiz, P. A., Lipsicas, C. B., Bobes, J., Cozman, D., Hegerl, U., & Zohar, J. (2016). Suicide prevention strategies revisited: 10-year systematic review. *The Lancet Psychiatry, 3*(7), 646–659. https://doi.org/10.1016/S2215-0366(16)30030-X

Chapter 9
Culturally Sensitive Suicide Prevention Programs: Addressing Indigenous Peoples in Latin America and the Caribbean

Marta Silva-Fernández and Belén Vargas

9.1 Suicide in Indigenous Communities of Latin America and the Caribbean

In Latin America and the Caribbean, understanding the phenomenon of suicide from an Indigenous perspective is critically important, as these regions comprise priority populations that are socially vulnerable and, therefore, more affected by suicide (World Health Organization, 2012). These populations are influenced by social determinants that constrain their socioeconomic position, leaving them in a significant situation of inequity (Irwin et al., 2006). Consequently, this region faces unique challenges characterized by cultural and social diversity, with Indigenous communities historically experiencing sociopolitical and territorial processes that directly impact their well-being.

It has been widely documented in international literature, in comparison to other continents, that suicide rates are elevated in many Indigenous populations worldwide. Pollock et al. (2018), in a systematic review of the global incidence of suicide in Indigenous populations, reported that in specific contexts, there is parity between Indigenous and non-Indigenous populations, while in other areas, rates are more than 20 times higher among Indigenous people. Similarly, Azuero et al. (2017), also

M. Silva-Fernández (✉)
Faculty of Philosophy and Humanities, Universidad Austral de Chile, Valdivia, Chile

Nucleus to Improve the Mental Health of Adolescents and Youths (Imhay), Santiago, Chile
e-mail: marta.silva@uach.cl

B. Vargas
Nucleus to Improve the Mental Health of Adolescents and Youths (Imhay), Santiago, Chile

Doctoral Program in Psychotherapy, Universidad de Chile and Pontificia Universidad Católica de Chile, Santiago, Chile

Mental Health Department, Ministerio de Salud, Santiago, Chile

Á. Jiménez-Molina, V. Martínez (eds.), *New Perspectives on Suicidal Behavior, Depression and Personality*, https://doi.org/10.1007/978-3-031-96037-6_9

in a systematic review, found that suicide rates are higher in the Indigenous population than in the non-Indigenous population and noted an increase in depression, anxiety, and other disorders within this population. These findings could be linked to what is known as "cultural death," a phenomenon in which changes in lifestyle, industrialization, degradation of the natural environment, and alcohol consumption become risk factors and triggers for suicide.

Recognition of inequality, racial discrimination, loss of land, and tensions in maintaining cultural identity are key elements in understanding this situation. A lack of attention to culturally specific perspectives in public policies for suicide prevention can perpetuate marginalization and fail to address the social determinants of mental health adequately. It is, therefore, imperative to move toward intercultural approaches that recognize and value cultural diversity, integrate Indigenous knowledge, and promote the active participation of these communities in decision-making.

Exploring and understanding the conceptions and meanings that different Latin American and Caribbean Indigenous cultures have about death and suicide, as well as assessing the current situation regarding policies and programs in this area, is one of the most important starting points for promoting culturally appropriate and effective policies and programs in this region, which needs further development in the field of mental health.

9.2 Meanings of the Phenomenon of Death in Indigenous Populations in Latin America

All human cultures assign a central place to the interpretation of the processes of human existence. Among these, the reproduction and representation of death and associated practices are fundamental aspects of cultural expression and understanding (Barnard & Spencer, 2010). The anthropology of death has traditionally studied death as a cultural phenomenon, a discipline concerned with the various ways in which human societies interpret, represent, and ritualize death and the dying process. The goal is to understand how different cultures make sense of the experience of loss, mourning, remembrance, and continuity of life and to analyze its social, political, economic, and religious implications (Duche, 2012).

Suicide from a cultural perspective has been studied in different Indigenous cultures, mainly in English-speaking countries (Azuero et al., 2017; Clifford et al., 2013; Pollock et al., 2018), but to a lesser extent in Indigenous populations in Latin America and the Caribbean. Existing studies in these regions have primarily focused on the phenomenon's epidemiology and its related factors from a Western biomedical perspective, as well as on preventive measures and interventions (Incayawar & Maldonado-Bouchard, 2009).

Thus, there is a need to explore the meanings that different Latin American and Caribbean cultures assign to death and suicide to incorporate them in the design of prevention policies. The concepts of death from different areas of Latin America will be presented to illustrate the similarities and differences in the beliefs. These examples will serve as a basis for understanding views on suicide and its related factors. Examples from Indigenous cultures in the Caribbean are not presented because of the scarcity of literature on suicide in these cultures in scholarly journals.

9.2.1 Indigenous Conceptions of Death

Indigenous cultures have unique conceptions of death that differ significantly from the Western notion of an absolute end. They understand death as a transition to another form of existence with a communal and relational sense of their worldview and nature.

Mesoamerican Náhuatl cultures do not perceive death as the end of life but as a cyclical continuation, a necessary dimension of the natural order, and a transformative process (Flores-Guerrero, 2011). The soul is believed to journey to the underworld, known as *mictlán*, where the person undergoes various trials. Rituals and ceremonies for the deceased guide and assist the soul in this journey (Johansson, 2014).

The Yukpa, who live in the Venezuelan valleys of the Sierra de Perijá, see death as a separation of the spiritual part of the person from the body, as in dreams or illness. They believe that physical death does not occur because the body stops functioning but because the spiritual parts are separated from the body forever. Hence, the lack of *yoramshi* or breath signals physical death and shows that the separation is permanent (Halbmayer, 2013).

For the Guaraní culture, located in the northeast of southern and southwestern Brazil, most of Paraguay, and southeastern Bolivia, death is referred to with the word *mano* and the expression *jehekýi*, which means to separate; that is, at death the soul is detached, separated from the body (Pozo, 2014). The Kaiowã and Nandeva (Both Guaranies cultures) communities believe in a connection between humans and the universe, where each element is under the guardianship of a guardian spirit called *Jara,* who is the owner of humanity (*ava Jara*). The highest deities of the Guaraní pantheon recognize two types of souls: the spiritual, introduced by the Nanderu in childhood, and the physical or shadow, which develops in adulthood. After death, the spiritual soul returns to the Guaraní sky, while the physical soul may wander near the place of death before moving on to a new abode in the southwest (*kururuy*). The progressive departure of the spirit soul may indicate illness caused by shamans or evil spirits, affecting the individual, family, and social ties. This phenomenon can become generalized, leading to *teko vai* (antisocial behavior) with behaviors such as aggression, violence, and rupture of family ties (Coloma et al., 2006).

The Aymara and Quechua Andean peoples, the former in the Chilean-Bolivian highlands and the latter in the highlands of Colombia, Ecuador, Peru, Bolivia, Argentina, and Chile, understand death as a natural part of life and as a continuity of existence, a transition to another plane. It has a collective and social dimension since the dead are part of the community, memory, and identity, as they are honored, remembered, and celebrated with rituals, offerings, songs, and dances. The person continues to exist and be present with the possibility of influencing the lives of the living (Flores & Abad, 2007). In funeral rituals, the community gathers to honor the deceased and support their journey to maintain a connection with the person and ensure their well-being. Reciprocity, a central concept in Andean cultures, is essential for the well-being of the living and the dead through rituals and offerings (van Kessel, 2001).

Further south in Latin America, the Mapuche culture of south-central Chile also sees death not as the end of life but as a transition to another plane facilitated by the *Machi*, a shaman who leads the *amulpüllún* ritual, which means "to make or force the soul or spirit to leave." It is a complex web of signs used to "speak" of death (Bacigalupo, 2014; Rojas, 2016). Thus, the *püllü* (soul) separates from the body to begin a condign journey, crossing a river and descending into the depths of the earth to penetrate the volcanoes to reach an island. The person must be packed with the food, liquid, and clothing he/she ate and wore when alive (Montecino, 1997). Likewise, the Pewenche of the Central-Southern Cordillera conceive of death as a gradual process, a journey to *kamapu* (other lands), where the dead have the freedom to travel through the cosmos, manifesting themselves in dreams and visions, giving advice and interceding before the spirits of life in favor of the people (Solar, 2013).

From the conceptions of death reviewed, common points can be identified. First, it is understood as a transition or continuation of existence on another plane, whether to the underworld, heaven, or other sacred lands, which is celebrated through rituals and ceremonies that pay homage to the deceased and guide them on their journey to maintain a connection with the person to ensure their well-being on the other plane. In addition, the deceased are believed to continue to be present and influence the lives of the living, emphasizing the importance of maintaining a relationship with them through rituals and offerings. Death takes on a collective and social dimension, bringing people together to ensure community and individual well-being.

9.2.2 Cultural Perspectives on Suicide and its Related Factors in the Yukpa-Irapa, Maya, Tikuna, Pai-Tavyterä, and Mapuche-Pehuenche Cultures

According to Corpas (2011), in the Yukpa-Irapa community of Venezuela, there is a strong relationship between imprisonment and the act of suicide. When faced with situations of incarceration, suicide is an immediate response to their problems. It would be an impulsive and unpremeditated act due to the emotional intensity of the moment. Several cases of suicide are directly related to the incarceration of a member of the community, making suicide a tool for resolving conflicts at both the personal and community levels. Suicide is seen as an act of courage. It also occurs in situations such as heartbreak or fear of abandonment by a partner, with death by one's hand being the most common solution (Corpas, 2011).

In Mayan culture, there was a specific deity associated with suicide called *Ixtab*, who guided people who died by suicide to the Mayan Paradise, a festive place with abundant food and drink, thus associating suicide with pleasure and joy and representing death by hanging. The Maya also believed in the existence of a giant tree called *ceiba* that was located in the center of the earth and acted as a link between the world of the living and the Mayan paradise; it symbolized release from suffering and misery and allowed those who die by suicide to ascend to higher levels (Casares, 2020; Damian, 2010; Mascayano et al., 2015; Singer, 2000). Suicide was not a directly voluntary act, as it could be provoked by various forms of evil known as *k'ok'o iik'* (bad wind) and *k'aak'as ba'al* (bad blood), which are malevolent spirits or predatory entities capable of influencing an individual's will and judgment or were interpreted as parts of the Mayan body. In the case of a hanging, these entities would come out of the body and attack family and community members. In addition (Ramírez, 2020), suicide could be the result of birthmarks that are considered omens or portents, such as the position of the umbilical cord around the neck of a newborn. Also, the *kuxa'an suum* (the living rope) could provoke this kind of death since it was used for hanging, but it is important to emphasize that it was not only an inert instrument. As its name suggests, the living rope had its agency. Other situations could lead to suicide among the Maya, such as *pu'ulyah* (witchcraft) or *xtáabay* (the spirit of a dead woman considered a monster) (Campbell, 2022; Ramírez, 2020).

In the Tikuna community of Nazareth, located on the Peruvian border with Colombia and Brazil, mental health is related to "being strong," meaning that spirits cannot enter their bodies to harm them or cause self-inflicted harm (Instituto Colombiano de Bienestar, 2020). Maintaining strength requires the guidance of traditional practitioners, who restore balance across the four pillars of Tikuna thought: *kṵa̰* (wisdom or knowledge), *pora* (power or strength), *naẽ* (thought), and *maü̃*. These elements ensure the preservation of culture (*pora*), participation and learning within their traditions (*naẽ*), the existence of the self (*maü̃*), and the transmission of accumulated knowledge (*kua̧*) (Velásquez, 2021). The loss of strength can be caused by the presence of jungle creatures, considered alert or risk factors because they endanger the community by taking away their will and leading them to self-destructive behaviors. An example is the Chachacuna, bearer of evil, who meets people and leads them to self-harm and suicide with knives, poison, or ropes. In this context, suicidal behavior is not perceived as the result of individual decisions but as the consequence of being under the influence of a third party. This spirit arises in response to negative emotions, thoughts, behaviors, or feelings (Instituto Colombiano de Bienestar, 2020).

In the Pai-tavyterä community, located in northwestern Paraguay, the concept of *tarujo* represents the leading cause that drives Pai Indians to decide suicide, considering it the best option at certain times. *Tarujo* is perceived as a disease sent by the gods that causes mental confusion and a state of hallucination in which voices are heard constantly harassing the sufferer, leading to an impulsive decision to suicide. Suicide is not socially accepted and is considered a negative way to die; those who choose this act follow a death ritual different from the rest of the people. They are buried in the same place where they ended their lives, rather than in a cemetery, and no ceremony is performed. There is also a belief that by choosing this way of dying, they will not receive any compensation in the afterlife (Corpas, 2011).

In southern Latin America, the Mapuche maintain that the concept of *küme monguen*, which is equivalent to "good living" in terms of well-being and health, is the result of a balance of harmonious reciprocal relationships between nature and humans and with the forces and beings that inhabit it. Nature is seen as a set of living forces that interact with man and reflect the balance of man in his community, called *lof*, and in its social, political, territorial, and religious dimensions. Any imbalance leads to a negative state known as *deweza felen*. According to Guajardo (2017), Western life in the twenty-first century makes it difficult to maintain this balance, and when the *che*, the person, becomes profoundly unbalanced, problems such as suicide, alcohol abuse, and domestic violence can occur. The act of suicide is attributed to *weda kurruf*, bad wind, and *Kalkutun,* evil, as hostile forces, with suicide being the result of a profound imbalance also caused by the modern Western lifestyle. An example of this was a wave of suicides and attempted suicides that occurred in the upper Biobío region of Chile during the installation of a hydroelectric dam in 2006–2007, which destroyed their ancestral territories. It is said that the *weda kurruf* came down the mountains, causing people to suicide due to the imbalance caused by the destruction of nature, which is reflected in the *che* (Guajardo, 2017; Parra et al., 2017).

Suicide is also explained in the Mapuche concept of duality, which states that good and evil manifest as energetic forces and spirits representing these two opposing spheres. Evil manifests itself in illnesses attributed to the actions of a *Kalku* (sorcerer) or someone endowed with this ability, usually motivated by envy or harmful desires toward another individual. When an act considered evil occurs in the community, it is recognized by its characteristics and manifests as a "kind of madness." A *Machi* must intervene; otherwise, the *kalkutun* may cause the person to suicide. Mistrustful relationships, competition, and disunity in the community aggravate the situation and increase the likelihood of experiencing a *kalkutun*, which may persist, suggesting the possibility that it will continue to affect more people (Guajardo, 2017).

The five presented and illustrative conceptions of suicide in Latin American Indigenous communities reveal some points of convergence. First, suicide goes beyond being an individual act and acquires a collective and communitarian dimension that affects the harmony and balance of these societies. Second, we can distinguish the spiritual and religious dimensions of suicide, where the explanations and meanings of suicide are derived from the beliefs, rites, myths, and symbols of each culture, influenced by supernatural forces. Finally, colonization, discrimination, violence, poverty, and loss of identity, especially those derived from territorial dispossession for resource extraction, emerge as recurrent external threats that contribute to mental and environmental imbalances and become key aspects of understanding this phenomenon (González-Parra & Simon, 2008; Ninomiya et al., 2023). Thus, suicide is revealed as a form of protest and resistance, sometimes collective, against intolerable situations, which is not only an act of despair but also an affirmation of identity reflected in the body as territory, that is, whatever happens on the earth (land) affects the body (MINSAL, 2016a, b). Thus, the causality of suicide goes beyond individual factors and recognizes the influence and confluence of the relational worldview and what colonization and modernity have brought.

9.3 Public Policies and Suicide Prevention

The development of public policies aimed at suicide prevention is of recent origin but is progressing rapidly. Considering that suicidal behavior is a significant public health problem, with high costs at the social and economic level for individuals and communities, in recent years, different countries have included in their policies different strategies to reduce mortality rates from this cause (Lewitzka et al., 2019). A notorious milestone was registered in the late 1990s when the World Health Organization (WHO) launched the global initiative Suicide Prevention—SUPRE to encourage the development of national suicide prevention strategies by member countries (World Health Organization, 2000). In 2013, suicide prevention was prioritized in the Mental Health Plan 2013–2020, adopted at the 66th WHO Assembly, which set a global target of a 10% reduction in suicide rates in countries by 2020 (World Health Organization, 2013). This was reinforced in 2014 with the iconic report "Preventing Suicide: A Global Imperative," which emphasized the need for a multisectoral approach to address suicide comprehensively (World Health Organization, 2014).

The inclusion of suicide mortality reduction as an indicator in the 2030 Agenda for Sustainable Development consolidates the issue as a global public policy area beyond the health sector. In the resolution signed by all United Nations member states, one of the goals is to reduce premature mortality from noncommunicable diseases by one-third by 2030, including through mental health promotion and prevention, and to include suicide prevention as a priority. (United Nations, 2015).

In 2014, only 28 countries reported developing some suicide prevention initiative (World Health Organization, 2014), rising to 62 countries six years later (World Health Organization, 2021b). Although this represents significant progress, it represents only about one-third of countries worldwide and is concentrated mainly in middle- and high-income countries.

The fact that a country has a national suicide prevention strategy means that it has systematically developed an integrated national response to this phenomenon, which has specific financial and human resources for its implementation. This implementation plan includes clear objectives, targets, indicators, and deadlines, along with designated responsibilities and concrete funding, so that evidence of its progress and/or impact can be monitored (World Health Organization, 2021a). What distinguishes a national strategy from individual prevention initiatives and programs is its multisectoral nature, which involves governments and constitutes a response to the problem following each country's cultural and social context (World Health Organization, 2012, 2018).

Suicide prevention policies should include different preventive components that provide a comprehensive response according to the multiple factors involved in the phenomenon. Likewise, policies should be designed with a multilevel approach, including specific interventions for those who have suicidal thoughts or behaviors, for those at higher risk, and the whole population. Components that are commonly found in national policies range from community awareness and education, epidemiological surveillance, and specific services to support people with lived experience of suicide, including treatment and postvention (Arensman, 2017; Platt et al., 2019; World Health Organization, 2014). A more detailed description of the usual components is provided in Table 9.1.

"LIVE LIFE," the WHO's latest guide to implementing suicide prevention policies, proposes distinguishing these components into cross-cutting core pillars and key effective interventions (World Health Organization, 2021a). Core pillars are the basis for the successful implementation of evidence-based interventions for suicide prevention, which are common to other public health policy areas. Key effective interventions are specific actions with proven effectiveness in suicide prevention that need to be implemented at the national level (Table 9.2).

In general, training, education, and surveillance are present in about 90% of existing strategies, while psychotherapy and crisis intervention are among the least implemented; the choice of components to prioritize in strategies may reflect the process in which each country is in policy development, as well as the influence of civil society, the participation of people with lived experience, and the willingness of countries to make prevention commitments. (Schlichthorst et al., 2023).

Public policies for suicide prevention need to be formulated considering not only individual risk factors but also those present at the macrosocial level, especially those that increase health inequalities and leave certain population groups more disadvantaged and vulnerable. Policies aimed at influencing the social determinants of health, such as improving living conditions and reducing discrimination and exclusion, should also be considered as part of national strategies to reduce suicidal behavior, benefiting not only those most at risk but the population as a whole; to move toward real integration of the different sectors in national prevention efforts, it is necessary to move toward a mental health vision in all policies and to overcome the barrier that restricts solutions to the health sector (Pirkis et al., 2023).

9.3.1 Suicide Prevention Policies and Indigenous Populations

In its successive publications, the WHO has emphasized that the most socially vulnerable populations are those most affected by suicide. Among them, Indigenous people are identified as one of the populations that nations should prioritize, supported by epidemiological evidence (World Health Organization, 2012). Within the higher risk of suicide for Indigenous people, social determinants converge that limit their socioeconomic position and leave them in a notorious situation of inequality (Irwin et al., 2006).

Table 9.1 Usual components of national suicide prevention strategies

Component	Target
Universal	
Restriction of access to means used for suicide	Reduce the availability, accessibility, and attractiveness of the means used for suicide (e.g., pesticides, firearms, high places). Reduce toxicity/lethality of available means.
Promotion of responsible media reporting	Promote the implementation of media guidelines for the responsible dissemination of suicide-related content in print, radio, television, and social media.
Awareness raising	Establish public information campaigns to support the understanding that suicides are preventable.
Addressing stigmatized attitudes toward mental ill-health and suicidal behavior	Increase public and professional access to information on all aspects of preventing suicidal behavior.
Surveillance, monitoring, and evaluation	Increase the quality and timeliness of national data on suicide and suicide attempts. Support establishing an integrated data collection system to identify vulnerable groups, individuals, and situations.
Oversight and coordination	Establish institutions or agencies to promote and coordinate research, training, and service delivery related to suicidal behavior. Strengthen the health and social system response to suicidal behavior.
Selective	
Access to health and social care services	Promote greater access to comprehensive health and social protection services for those vulnerable to suicidal behavior.
Training and education	Develop or strengthen competencies for the detection, first response, and care of people at risk of suicide, both at the community and health team levels (e.g., gatekeepers in the community, primary health care personnel, mental health providers).
Indicated	
Psychotherapeutic interventions intended to reduce repeated suicidal behavior	Improve the quality of health care and evidence-based clinical interventions, especially for people presenting to emergency departments after a suicide attempt. Improve research and evaluation of effective interventions.
Enhanced care/follow-up targeted at people with a history of attempted suicide	Registration in emergency departments of persons who have attempted suicide. Continuity of care through telephone follow-up of people who have attempted suicide and provision of brief counseling. Encouraging people who have attempted suicide to use mental health services.
Crisis intervention	Ensure that communities respond to crises with appropriate interventions and that people in a crisis can access emergency mental health care, including through hotlines or the Internet.
Postvention	Improve response and care for people affected by suicide and suicide attempts, including support and recovery services.

Note: Based on Platt et al. (2019) and World Health Organization (2014, 2021a)

Indigenous participation in policy formulation is the primary strategy proposed by the WHO. This participation can be expressed by including Indigenous representatives and leaders as part of consultative councils and in decision-making at different organizational levels, from national policies to territorial definitions (World Health Organization, 2012, 2018).

Table 9.2 Core components of LIVE LIFE approach

Cross-cutting core pillars	Key effective interventions
Situation analysis Multisectoral collaboration Awareness-raising and advocacy Capacity-building Financing Surveillance, monitoring, and evaluation	Limit access to the means of suicide. Interact with the media for responsible reporting of suicide. Foster socio-emotional life skills in adolescents. Early identify, assess, manage, and follow up anyone who is affected by suicidal behaviors.

Note: Based on World Health Organization (2021a)

On the other hand, one of the most critical aspects is to find ways to incorporate specific strategies for Indigenous peoples in public policies without maintaining the status quo of the supremacy of the Western model over Indigenous systems. The field of suicide prevention has been discussed as being based on a biomedical and individual-centered model and, therefore, culturally misaligned with Indigenous paradigms of health, mental wellness, and a collective outlook (Fitzpatrick et al., 2015). According to this view, the development of public policies for Indigenous peoples must begin with a contextualized vision of what suicide means, which generates the basis for the design of tailored strategies and overcomes a homogeneous vision of the phenomenon and the solutions to prevent it; therefore, the goal of merely adapting strategies to people's cultural reality is insufficient and even comparable to a new exercise in cultural assimilation (Anderson, 2021).

Initiatives based on holistic processes of engaging with culture and strengthening connectedness, integrating Indigenous knowledge, and using decolonizing approaches have been shown to have an impact on suicide-related outcomes at the individual and community levels, as evidenced by experiences in Indigenous populations in Canada, the United States, Australia, and New Zealand (Sjoblom et al., 2022).

The New Agenda for Mental Health in the Americas, which identifies ten immediate priorities for mental health policy in the wake of COVID-19, includes suicide prevention as one of them and adds addressing racial discrimination as one of the most important social determinants of mental health in the region. It calls for combating systemic racism against Indigenous peoples, as well as other ethnic and racial minorities, through environmental interventions, the formulation of national plans against racism, and legislation (PAHO, 2023). This is undoubtedly a significant step forward but needs governments' commitment.

9.4 Lessons from Latin America and the Caribbean

The WHO systematically maps mental health resources worldwide through the Mental Health Atlas project. It provides an up-to-date overview of the profiles of mental health systems in different countries and regions. Its latest version provides an overview of the implementation of national suicide prevention initiatives or programs. Specifically for Latin America and the Caribbean, of the 28 countries that provided information, only 18 reported the existence of a national suicide prevention strategy (World Health Organization, 2021b).

After reviewing the public documents on the various strategies that make up public policy on suicide prevention, four of the 18 countries stand out, including specific considerations related to Indigenous populations: Brazil, Chile, Colombia, Costa Rica, and Ecuador. A common aspect that can be seen in these experiences is the declaration as a starting point of the recognition of the existence of socio-political processes in the region that have directly affected the different Indigenous populations, such as the loss of land, social marginalization, poverty, tensions in the preservation of cultural identity, and the risk of cultural and physical survival or extinction of Indigenous communities.

The proposals made by the countries to direct preventive efforts to these groups can be grouped into four thematic areas, described below.

9.4.1 Explicit Recognition in Policy Formulation

This involves the recognition of Indigenous peoples as a priority population group. From a political perspective, this action involves a gesture of visibility for a historically excluded group. It opens the door to generating specific targets and initiatives within a macropolicy.

Countries can materialize recognition in different ways and to different degrees. The first form is the designation of Indigenous peoples as a group for which it is necessary to develop selective strategies. An example is what Colombia is doing as part of its National Suicide Prevention Strategy (Ministry of Health and Social Protection, 2021). The Strategy recognizes the urgent need to address suicidal behavior in Indigenous populations. The Strategy proposes a series of key actions that can be implemented to effectively address this problem, including, for example, intersectoral and intercultural participatory actions with a community focus and raising awareness among the population on issues such as racism, discrimination, and prejudice.

The formalization of recognition can be concretized through defining specific goals in public policy. For example, Brazil's Agenda of Strategic Actions for Suicide Surveillance and Prevention and Health Promotion 2017–2020 includes an objective to "recognize the specificity of suicide among Indigenous peoples in the planning and implementation of strategic actions related to the issue" (p. 13). This commitment stems from the recognition that the rate of suicide among Indigenous peoples is approximately twice that of the general population and that this has a significant impact on Indigenous communities, affecting not only the individuals who die from this cause but also their families and communities (Ministério da Saúde, 2017).

It is important to emphasize that when prioritizing Indigenous groups in policies, it should be explained that intrinsic individual characteristics do not mainly give the risk, but rather by the interaction that occurs between different factors and the person, where vulnerability is more significant in the face of recurrent exposure to situations of violence and discrimination, which translates into experiences of chronic stress, stigmatization, social exclusion, and economic disadvantage (MINSAL, 2019).

9.4.2 Incorporating Culturally Sensitive Approaches

The integration of culturally sensitive approaches into suicide prevention policies is fundamental to addressing inequities and ensuring the right to health of Indigenous peoples. The intercultural approach to health has been promoted in the Region of the Americas as a response to address inequities and ensure the right to health, advocating for the recognition and respect of different cultural groups, the integration of their knowledge systems, and participation in health care (PAHO, 2019).

Five aspects are central to the intercultural approach in policy: (1) recognition and appreciation of cultural diversity; (2) collaboration with traditional medicine and integration of ancestral health practices into health systems; (3) active participation of communities in decision-making about their health, ensuring an inclusive and respectful perspective; (4) cultural sensitivity in health care; (5) elimination of health inequalities, ensuring that all people, regardless of their cultural background, have access to quality health services (PAHO/World Health Organization, 2017). An intercultural approach to health enables countries to fulfill the right to provide health services that respect people's cultures (UN, 2000).

Incorporating an intercultural approach in suicide prevention policies can be realized through affirmative action to close gaps and inequalities (Ministry of Public Education, 2018). Also, through the strengthening of cultural practices specific to each Indigenous people, the rescue of ancestral knowledge and the use of community networks available for collective support of people affected by suicide or mental illness, as well as the joint definition with Indigenous authorities and traditional knowledgeable people of the path that should include intercultural health care (Ministry of Health and Social Protection, 2021).

The application of an intercultural approach in the design of public policies for suicide prevention implies the establishment of horizontal and reciprocal relations with Indigenous cultural systems in the design and implementation of public policies, based on the recognition of inequalities and power asymmetries and the cultural dominance exercised by Western paradigms transferred to the health system.

9.4.3 Data Collection and Epidemiologic Surveillance

Data collection and epidemiological surveillance disaggregated by Indigenous peoples are essential to understanding and addressing suicide in these communities. Examples such as that of Ecuador, which disaggregates information by ethnicity, have made it possible to identify significant differences in the lethal methods used by specific Indigenous populations, such as the Waoranis and Shuar (Ministry of Public Health of Ecuador, 2021). For its part, Brazil proposes the inclusion of variables related to suicide risk in population surveys and information systems, focusing on priority groups (Ministério da Saúde, 2017).

In Chile, the disaggregation of data allowed for elaborating differentiated epidemiological profiles for different Indigenous populations in specific geographic areas, identifying health gaps, and designing culturally sensitive and geographically localized policies and programs. These analyses have confirmed the higher risk of death by suicide among Indigenous people in different regions of the country and different Indigenous groups; they have revealed a recurrent pattern of higher risk of death by suicide among Indigenous people under 30 years of age, male and living in rural areas (MINSAL, 2006, 2008, 2009, 2011, 2012; MINSAL & CEPAL, 2009, 2010). In addition, progress has been made in incorporating diversity in information systems and the production and availability of data disaggregated by Indigenous affiliation by including them in the minimum and obligatory set of personal data in the standards of health information records (MINSAL, 2018). This has made it possible to identify the Indigenous population that consults the different points of care of the public health system for reasons related to suicidal ideation or suicidal behavior (MINSAL, 2023).

The disaggregation of data by Indigenous populations provides opportunities to monitor and evaluate the effectiveness of specific suicide prevention interventions in these communities. This is essential for adapting and continuously improving prevention and treatment strategies.

9.4.4 Strengthening Cultural Competence in Health Care Teams

Intercultural competence in health care teams is essential to ensure effective and appropriate work with people from different cultural contexts. These competencies include the knowledge, skills, and attitudes needed to understand how other cultural groups see and interpret the world and facilitate interaction between the healthcare team and the population served. In addition, they include awareness of one's own biases and preconceptions about cultural groups other than one's own (Alizadeh & Chavan, 2016), recognizing that the Western medical system is one of the possible interpretations of reality that coexist today (MINSAL, 2016a, b).

Based on intercultural competence, it is possible to create health interventions that are ethical and equitable when it comes to cross-cultural encounters (Henderson et al., 2018). Lack of cultural competence in mental health teams and services can lead to mistrust and alienation of people in need of care (Griner & Smith, 2006), which in turn creates an entirely avoidable barrier to health access, that is, health inequity. Capacity building in the health sector also allows for the socio-cultural adaptation of intervention guidelines according to each territorial reality (Ministry of Health and Social Protection, 2006).

Efforts to provide technical guidance to health teams to develop greater cultural competence and to implement culturally relevant suicide prevention interventions in Indigenous communities are highlighted. A common aspect seen in Latin American countries developing in this area is the elaboration of technical guidelines with the participation of Indigenous representatives and the collection of successful experiences from the health teams themselves. An example of this is the technical guidelines developed in Brazil (Ministério da Saúde, 2019), Chile (MINSAL, 2016a, b) and Colombia (MINSALUD, 2016). Another example is the training manual for community caregivers in Ecuador (Ministry of Public Health, 2019), which provides guidelines for suicide prevention training for Indigenous community agents.

9.5 Toward Culturally Sensitive Suicide Prevention

From the review of cultural conceptions of death, suicide, and its causality, and then on suicide prevention policies in Indigenous populations in Latin America and the Caribbean, the urgent need to address suicide in Indigenous communities from an intercultural approach in prevention and postvention policies with an interdisciplinary perspective in health sciences is highlighted, especially with the decline in the composition and professional training of teams of health professionals working with Indigenous groups. The adoption of transversal policies should go beyond individual factors; one of the central pillars of the political and social dynamics that influence the problem of suicide should be established, such as the destruction of ecosystems, which due to their constitutive and relational nature, in the words of Urrego-Mendoza (2017) "For Indigenous peoples, losing the territory is like death, it is stripping its essence, altering the balance, detaching it from the mother; 'without territory, there is no life'. To leave an Indigenous person without territory is to condemn them to physical and cultural extermination."

The design and implementation of policies should adopt integrative perspectives between the biomedical model and Indigenous worldviews concerning the risk factors in which they find themselves (destruction of ecosystems, isolation, and discrimination, among others), allowing the implementation of culturally relevant interventions. Understanding and addressing suicide in Indigenous populations in Latin America, as well as in the world, must go beyond the limits of Western epidemiology,

Recognition of this complexity suggests the adoption of strategies based on Western holistic theoretical models and Indigenous epistemologies—methods of inquiry to co-design suicide prevention policies with Indigenous groups themselves. These strategies may include, for example, the application of Bronfenbrenner's ecological model, as well as Indigenous epistemological conceptions and research methodologies, such as talking circles, dialogues with elders, healing rituals, and the incorporation of the concept of "good life" found in several Latin American cultures (Carreño-Calderón, 2021; Marsh et al., 2016), together with biomedical models to develop interventions developed by the communities themselves. This would allow us to cover the phenomenon from a micro perspective, considering individual and family factors, to a macroperspective, examining the social, cultural, and political influences that contribute to the phenomenon. All this is in a context in which the Indigenous communities' knowledge becomes the main framework for developing effective and culturally sensitive strategies to promote the mental health and well-being of these populations.

Acknowledgments This manuscript was supported by ANID—Millennium Science Initiative Program NCS2021_081 and by ANID—FONDECYT N° 1242006. BV received funding from ANID/BECA DOCTORADO NACIONAL/2021_21212114.

References

Alizadeh, S., & Chavan, M. (2016). Cultural competence dimensions and outcomes: A systematic review of the literature. *Health & Social Care in the Community, 24*(6), e117–e130. https://doi.org/10.1111/hsc.12293

Anderson, B. (2021). The structural violence of indigenous suicide prevention policies in Canada. *Anthropology in Action, 28*(3), 22–34. https://doi.org/10.3167/aia.2021.280303

Arensman, E. (2017). Suicide prevention in an international context. *Crisis, 38*(1), 1–6. https://doi.org/10.1027/0227-5910/a000461

Azuero, A. J., Arreaza-Kaufman, D., Coriat, J., Tassinari, S., Faria, A., Castañeda-Cardona, C., & Rosselli, D. (2017). Suicide in the indigenous population of Latin America: A systematic review. *Revista colombiana de psiquiatria, 46*(4), 237–242. https://doi.org/10.1016/j.rcp.2016.12.002

Bacigalupo, A. M. (2014). The potency of indigenous "bibles" and biographies: Mapuche shamanic literacy and historical consciousness. *American Ethnologist, 41*(4), 648–663. https://doi.org/10.1111/amet.12103

Barnard, A., & Spencer, J. (Eds.). (2010). *The Routledge encyclopedia of social and cultural anthropology*. Routledge.

Bronfenbrenner, U. (1979). *The ecology of human development*. Harvard University Press.

Campbell, S. (2022). The xtáabay as monstrous woman. *Monsters in Performance*, 61–70. https://doi.org/10.4324/9781003137337-6

Carreño-Calderón, A. (2021). Living well and health practices among aymara people in northern Chile. *Latin American Perspectives, 48*(3), 69–81. https://doi.org/10.1177/0094582x211004908

Clifford, A. C., Doran, C. M., & Tsey, K. (2013). A systematic review of suicide prevention interventions targeting indigenous peoples in Australia, United States, Canada and New Zealand. *BMC Public Health, 13*, 1–11.

Coloma, C., Hoffman, J. S., & Crosby, A. (2006). Suicide among Guaraní Kaiowá and Nandeva Youth in Mato Grosso do Sul, Brazil. *Archives of Suicide Research, 10*(2), 191–207. https://doi.org/10.1080/13811110600662505

Colombian Institute of Family Welfare. (2020). *Suicidal behavior in indigenous children, adolescents and youth of Nazareth, Amazonas: Guidelines for prevention and care*. Team National University of Colombia – Amazonian Headquarters.

Corpas, J. M. (2011). Social and cultural approach to the phenomenon of suicide. Amerindian ethnic communities. *Gazeta de Antropología, 27*(2).

Damian, C. (2010). *Domination without dominance: Inca-Spanish encounters in early colonial Peru*. Duke University.

Duche, A. (2012). The anthropology of death: Authors, approaches and periods. *Society and Religion, 37*, 2006–2215.

Fitzpatrick, S. J., Hooker, C., & Kerridge, I. (2015). Suicidology as a social practice. *Social Epistemology, 29*(3), 303–322. https://doi.org/10.1080/02691728.2014.895448

Flores, J. A., & Abad, L. (2007). *Ethnographies of death and cultures in Latin America*. University of Castilla La Mancha.

Flores-Guerrero, R. (2011). Health, illness and death: Readings from sociocultural anthropology. *MAD Journal, 0*(10). https://doi.org/10.5354/0718-0527.2004.14783

González-Parra, C., & Simon, J. (2008). All that glitters is not gold: Resettlement, vulnerability, and social exclusion in the Pehuenche community Ayin Mapu, Chile. *American Behavioral Scientist, 51*(12), 1774–1789.

Griner, D., & Smith, T. B. (2006). Culturally adapted mental health intervention: A meta-analytic review. *Psychotherapy: Theory, Research, Practice, Training, 43*(4), 531–548. https://doi.org/10.1037/0033-3204.43.4.531

Guajardo, G. (Ed.). (2017). *Contemporary suicides: Links, inequalities and socio-cultural transformations. Essays on violence, culture and meaning*. FLACSO-Chile.

Halbmayer, E. (2013). Securing a Life for the Dead among the Yukpa. The exhumation ritual as a temporary synchronisation of worlds. *Journal de la Société des Américanistes, 99*(1), 105–140. https://doi.org/10.4000/jsa.12620

Henderson, S., Horne, M., Hills, R., & Kendall, E. (2018). Cultural competence in healthcare in the community: A concept analysis. *Health & Social Care in the Community, 26*(4), 590–603. https://doi.org/10.1111/hsc.12556

Incayawar, M., & Maldonado-Bouchard, S. (2009). The forsaken mental health of the Indigenous Peoples-a moral case of outrageous exclusion in Latin America. *BMC International Health and Human Rights, 9*, 1–5. https://doi.org/10.1186/1472-698X-9-27

Irwin, A., Valentine, N., Brown, C., Loewenson, R., Solar, O., Brown, H., Koller, T., & Vega, J. (2006). The commission on social determinants of health: Tackling the social roots of health inequities. *PLoS Medicine, 3*(6), 749–751. https://doi.org/10.1371/journal.pmed.0030106

Johansson, K. (2014). Nenomamictiliztli: Suicide in the pre-Hispanic Nahuatl world. *Studies in Nahuatl culture, 47*, 53–119.

Lewitzka, U., Sauer, C., Bauer, M., & Felber, W. (2019). Are national suicide prevention programs effective? A comparison of 4 verum and 4 control countries over 30 years. *BMC Psychiatry, 19*(1), 158. https://doi.org/10.1186/s12888-019-2147-y

Marsh, T. N., Cote-Meek, S., Young, N. L., Najavits, L. M., & Toulouse, P. (2016). Indigenous healing and seeking safety: A blended implementation project for intergenerational trauma and substance use disorders. *The International Indigenous Policy Journal, 7*(2).

Mascayano, F., Irrazabal, M., Emilia, W. D., Vaner, S. J., Sapag, J. C., Alvarado, R., Yang, L. H., & Sinah, B. (2015). Suicide in Latin America: A growing public health issue. *Revista de la Facultad de Ciencias Medicas, 72*(4), 295–303.

Ministry of Health. (2017). *Agenda de Ações Estratégicas para a Vigilância e Prevenção do Suicídio e Promoção da Saúde no Brasil*. Ministério da Saúde, Secretaria de Atenção à Saúde, Departamento de Ações Programáticas Estratégicas.

Ministry of Health. (2019). *Estratégias de Prevenção do Suicídio em Povos Indígenas. Ministério da Saúde. Secretaria Especial de Saúde Indígena*. Departamento de Atenção à Saúde Indígena. https://bvsms.saude.gov.br/bvs/publicacoes/Estrategia_Prevencao_Suicidio_Povos_Indigenas.pdf.

Ministry of Health and Social Protection. (2021). *National Strategy for the Prevention of Suicidal Behavior in Colombia*. Ministry of Health and Social Protection. https://www.minsalud.gov.co/sites/rid/Lists/BibliotecaDigital/RIDE/VS/PP/ENT/estrategia-nacional-conducta-suicida-2021.pdf

Ministry of Public Education. (2018). *Protocol of attention to the student population presenting self-inflicted injuries and/or at risk for suicide attempts*. Ministry of Public Education, Directorate of Student Life. https://psicologosemergenciasbaleares.files.wordpress.com/2022/01/protocolo-prevencion-suicidio.pdf.

Ministry of Public Health. (2019). *Training for community caregivers on suicide. Manual. Dirección Nacional de Normatización - MSP*. https://www.salud.gob.ec/wp-content/uploads/2021/09/Manual-de-prevencion-del-suicidio_06-09-2021_MSP.pdf.

MINSAL. (2006). *Basic epidemiological profile of the Aymara population of the Arica Health Service*. Ministry of Health, Chile.

MINSAL. (2008). *Basic epidemiological profile of the mapuche population. Communes of the lafkenche area of the Araucanía Sur Health Service*. Ministry of Health, Chile.

MINSAL. (2009). *Basic epidemiological profile. Kawésqar, Yámana and Mapuche-williche peoples. Magallanes Region*. Ministry of Health, Chile.

MINSAL. (2011). *Basic epidemiological profile of the Mapuche population residing in the coverage area of the Araucanía Norte Health Service*. Ministry of Health, Chile.

MINSAL. (2012). *Serie análisis de la situación de salud de los pueblos indígenas de Chile, N° 9. Perfil epidemiológico básico de la población mapuche residente en el área de cobertura del Servicio de Salud Osorno*. Ministerio de Salud, Chile.

MINSAL. (2016a). *Orientaciones técnicas para la atención de salud mental con pueblos indígenas: Hacia un enfoque intercultural*. Subsecretaria de Salud Pública/Subsecretaria de Redes Asistenciales, Ministerio de Salud, Chile.

MINSAL. (2016b). *Technical guidelines for mental health care with Indigenous Peoples: Towards an intercultural approach*. Subsecretaría de Salud Pública, Subsecretaría de Redes Asistenciales. Ministerio de Salud, Chile.

MINSAL. (2018). *Technical guidelines cultural relevance in health information systems. Variable of Belonging to Indigenous Peoples in the Health Sector Statistical Records and Forms*. Ministerio de Salud, Chile.

MINSAL. (2019). *Recommendations for the prevention of suicidal behavior in educational establishments. Development of preventive strategies for School Communities*. National Suicide Prevention Program, Ministry of Health, Chile.

MINSAL. (2023). *Reportería Programa de Salud Mental*. https://informesdeis.minsal.cl/SASVisualAnalytics/?reportUri=%2Freports%2Freports%2Fad0c03ad-ee7a-4das4-bcc7-73d6e12920cf&sectionIndex=0&sso_guest=true&reportViewOnly=true&sas-welcome=false

MINSAL & CEPAL. (2009). *Basic epidemiological profile of the Mapuche population residing in the Los Ríos Region*. Ministry of Health.

MINSAL & CEPAL. (2010). *Basic epidemiological profile of the plan population residing in Arauco Province*. Ministry of Health.

MINSALUD. (2016). *Technical guidelines with intercultural approach for the promotion of mental health, prevention of psychoactive substance use and suicidal behavior in indigenous population*. Directorate of Promotion and Prevention Subdirectorate of Noncommunicable Diseases. Ministry of Health and Social Protection. https://www.minsalud.gov.co/sites/rid/Lists/BibliotecaDigital/RIDE/VS/PP/ENT/salud-mental-indigena-orientaciones-tecnicas.pdf

Montecino, S. (1997). The river of tears. *Anales de la Universidad de Chile, 6*, 1–17.

PAHO. (2019). *Strategy and plan of action on ethnicity and health 2019–2025*. Pan American Health Organization. https://iris.paho.org/bitstream/handle/10665.2/51744/PAHOEGC19002_eng.pdf?sequence=1&isAllowed=y

PAHO. (2023). *A new agenda for mental health in the Americas: Report of the Pan American Health Organization High-Level Commission on Mental Health and COVID-19*. Pan American Health Organization.

PAHO/World Health Organization. (2017). *Policy on ethnicity and health (29th Pan American Sanitary Conference)*. https://www.paho.org/es/documentos/politica-sobre-etnicidad-salud-29a-conferencia-sanitaria-panamericana.

Parra, C. G., Simon, J. W., & Jara, E. (2017). Etiologies of Pehuenche suicide: Territorial trauma and negative forces in Alto Biobío, Chile. In G. Guajardo (Ed.), *Contemporary suicides: Bonds, inequalities, and sociocultural transformations. Essays on violence, culture and meaning*. FLACSO.

Pirkis, J., Gunnell, D., Hawton, K., Hetrick, S., Niederkrotenthaler, T., Sinyor, M., Yip, P. S. F., & Robinson, J. (2023). A public health, whole-of-government approach to national suicide prevention strategies. *Crisis, 44*(2), 85–92. https://doi.org/10.1027/0227-5910/a000902

Platt, S., Arensman, E., & Rezaeian, M. (2019). National suicide prevention strategies – progress and challenges. *Crisis, 40*(2), 75–82. https://doi.org/10.1027/0227-5910/a000587

Pollock, J., Naicker, K., Loro, A., et al. (2018). Global incidence of suicide among Indigenous peoples: A systematic review. *BMC Medicine, 16*, 2–17. https://doi.org/10.1186/s12916-018-1115-6

Pozo, M. (2014). *Social representations about death in villages originating in the province of Jujuy*. Dissemination. Catholic University of Santiago del Estero. UCSE Editions.

Ramírez, M. A. (2020). Of violence and stereotypes. Visions around suicidal death in Yucatecan Mayan populations. *Estudios de historia moderna y contemporánea de México, 60*, 79–110.

Rojas, P. (2016). The Mapuche funeral rite of rest: From ontological moulting to the tree of the ancestors. *Chungará, 48*(4), 657–678. https://doi.org/10.4067/S0717-73562016005000023

Schlichthorst, M., Reifels, L., Spittal, M., Clapperton, A., Scurrah, K., Kolves, K., Platt, S., Pirkis, J., & Krysinska, K. (2023). Evaluating the effectiveness of components of national suicide prevention strategies. *Crisis, 44*(4), 318–328. https://doi.org/10.1027/0227-5910/a000887

Singer, M. O. (2000). Under the shadow of the great ceiba: The cosmovision of the Lacandones. *Desacatos, 5*, 45–56.

Sjoblom, E., Ghidei, W., Leslie, M., James, A., Bartel, R., Campbell, S., & Montesanti, S. (2022). Centering Indigenous knowledge in suicide prevention: A critical scoping review. *BMC Public Health, 22*(1), 2377. https://doi.org/10.1186/s12889-022-14580-0

Solar, T. L. (2013). *Morte pela própria mão: Estudo etnográfico de narrativas dos Mapuche Pewenche do Alto Bío Bío, no Chile, sobre suicídios acontecidos nas comunidades* [Master's thesis]. Federal University of Santa Catarina. https://repositorio.ufsc.br/handle/123456789/106796

United Nations. (2015). *Transforming our world: The 2030 agenda for sustainable development* (A/RES/70/1). https://sustainabledevelopment.un.org/post2015/transformingourworld/publication

United Nations (UN). (2000). *Committee on Economic, Social and Cultural Rights (CESCR), General Comment No 14 (2000): The right to the highest attainable standard of health (article 12 of the International Covenant on Economic, Social and Cultural Rights)*, 11 August 2000, E/C.12/2000/4.

Urrego-Mendoza, Z., Bastidas-Jacanamijoy, M., Coral-Palchucán, G., & Bastidas-Jacanamijoy, L. (2017). Narrativas sobre la conducta suicida en pueblos indígenas colombianos, 1993–2013. *Revista Facultad Nacional de Salud Pública, 35*(3), 400–409.

Van Kessel, J. (2001). The mortuary ritual of the Aymara of Tarapacá as experience and nurturing of life. *Chungará, 33*(2), 221–234. https://doi.org/10.4067/s0717-73562001000200006

Velásquez, O. (2021). *Desarrollo y suicidio de indígenas tikuna en Leticia y Puerto Nariño, Amazonas: Un análisis desde la decolonialidad y el postdesarrollo*. Universidad de Los Andes.

World Health Organization. (2000). *Preventing suicide a resource for primary health care workers*. World Health Organization.

World Health Organization. (2012). *Public health action for the prevention of suicide: A framework*. World Health Organization. https://iris.who.int/handle/10665/75166

World Health Organization. (2013). *Mental health action plan 2013–2020*. World Health Organization. https://www.who.int/publications-detail-redirect/9789241506021

World Health Organization. (2014). *Preventing suicide: A global imperative*. World Health Organization.

World Health Organization. (2018). *National suicide prevention strategies: Progress, examples and indicators*. World Health Organization. https://iris.who.int/handle/10665/279765

World Health Organization. (2021a). *Live life: An implementation guide for suicide prevention in countries*. World Health Organization.

World Health Organization. (2021b). *Mental Health Atlas 2020*. World Health Organization. https://iris.who.int/bitstream/handle/10665/345946/9789240036703-eng.pdf?sequence=1

Chapter 10
Suicide Bereavement and Postvention: What Do We Know and What Should We Know?

Álvaro Jiménez-Molina, Francisco Ojeda Güemes, Thiare Barrera, Juan Pablo Pinto, and Margot Morgiève

10.1 The Aftermath of Suicide

A significant number of people will face the loss of a loved one or acquaintance to suicide at some point in their lives. Although it is difficult to estimate the exact number of individuals exposed to a suicide death, roughly one in twenty people will experience this within a year and one in five throughout their lifetime (Andriessen et al., 2017). A study estimated that the lifetime prevalence of losing a family member to suicide is 3.9%, while the prevalence of losing a friend is 14.5% (Andriessen et al., 2017). Another study revealed that approximately 51% of the general population knew someone who had died by suicide, and 35% of these individuals reported feeling affected by the loss (Feigelman et al., 2018). Additionally, it is estimated that each suicide can affect between six and 135 individuals, with some experiencing a profound impact (Cerel et al., 2019; McDonnell et al., 2022).

The term "suicide survivors" refers to individuals who have lost a loved one or close person to suicide and have been affected by this loss to varying degrees or whose lives have changed as a result (Cerel et al., 2014). Losing someone to suicide

Á. Jiménez-Molina (✉)
Faculty of Psychology and Humanities, Universidad San Sebastián,
Santiago, RM - Santiago, Chile

Millennium Institute for Research in Depression and Personality (MIDAP), Santiago, Chile

Nucleus to Improve the Mental Health of Adolescents and Youths (Imhay), Santiago, Chile
e-mail: alvaro.jimenez@uss.cl

F. Ojeda Güemes
Faculty of Psychology and Humanities, Universidad San Sebastián, Santiago, Chile

T. Barrera · J. P. Pinto
Faculty of Psychology, Universidad Diego Portales, Santiago, Chile

M. Morgiève
CERMES3, Inserm, Université Paris Cité, Paris, France

Á. Jiménez-Molina, V. Martínez (eds.), *New Perspectives on Suicidal Behavior*, Depression and Personality, https://doi.org/10.1007/978-3-031-96037-6_10

is a significant risk factor for mental health problems, yet those grieving a suicide loss often do not receive the necessary support (Ross et al., 2021). Furthermore, they frequently encounter barriers in accessing professional support, as healthcare providers may not always know where to refer them (Wainwright et al., 2020).

The recognition of the significant impact of suicide is reflected in the increased research on suicide bereavement over the past two decades (Maple et al., 2018), highlighting the growing need to develop and implement "postvention" strategies.

Like universal, selective, and indicated interventions—designed to address social and individual risk factors, as well as those already at risk of suicide—the term "postvention" refers to a set of supportive and assistance actions aimed at individuals and communities after a suicide. The primary goal of postvention is to accompany affected individuals, families, or communities to facilitate the grieving process, allow for the healthy expression of the suffering caused by the loss, and promote recovery or stabilization of everyday life after suicide (Andriessen et al., 2019a, b). Additionally, postvention seeks to prevent further suicidal behaviors among other affected family or community members. Thus, postvention can be seen as a form of selective or indicated intervention, as those who have lost a loved one to suicide face an increased risk of suicide themselves (Hill et al., 2020).

This chapter provides an overview of the current knowledge on suicide bereavement and postvention. It examines the characteristics of the suicide bereavement process and describes various support strategies for survivors, including mutual support groups and programs implemented in different settings (community, healthcare services, schools). Finally, it addresses key challenges in research and postvention interventions.

10.2 Understanding Suicide Bereavement

The loss of a loved one to suicide disrupts the everyday lives of individuals, potentially having severe consequences for physical and mental health, as well as the well-being of families and communities for a considerable time (McDonnell et al., 2022; Pitman et al., 2014). The varying levels of impact suicide has on people have been described as the "continuum of survivorship" (Cerel et al., 2014). This model suggests an impact range from being "exposed" (anyone who knows someone who has died by suicide), to being "affected" (experiencing distress but not considering oneself in mourning), or "bereaved" by suicide (a significant short- or long-term impact due to the death).

Suicide bereavement refers to the process of grief and adjustment experienced by family members, friends, and close contacts following the death of a loved one by suicide (Pitman et al., 2014). Although the adverse health effects can depend on the closeness to the deceased, those affected by suicide are not limited to close family or friends but also include broader networks such as educational and work environments and healthcare professionals (Maple et al., 2018; McDonnell et al., 2022).

Compared to the general population, survivors suffer negative effects on eating and sleeping habits, have a higher risk of physical illnesses such as cardiovascular diseases, and are two to three times more likely to experience mental health problems (De Groot & Kollen, 2013; Pitman et al., 2014; McDonnell et al., 2022), including depressive and anxiety disorders, post-traumatic stress disorder, and a higher likelihood of psychiatric hospitalization (Cerel et al., 2014; Pitman et al., 2014; Mitchell & Terhorst, 2017).

Exposure to suicide and the grief associated with it also contribute to a heightened risk of suicidal behavior (Hill et al., 2020). A study conducted in the United Kingdom shows that adults bereaved by suicide were 65% more likely to attempt suicide than those grieving sudden natural causes (Pitman et al., 2016). It is estimated that nearly 10% of individuals bereaved by suicide subsequently attempt suicide. Unlike the typical gender gap in suicidality, suicide attempts occur in similar proportions among male and female survivors (McDonnell et al., 2022). A systematic review and meta-analysis examined the relationship between exposure to various forms of suicidal behavior (suicide, suicide attempts, and suicidal ideation) and their subsequent effects (Hill et al., 2020). The findings revealed that exposure to suicide increases the risk of both suicide and suicide attempts, with no significant association found with suicidal ideation. The death of a family member by suicide triples an individual's odds of attempting suicide, while the death of a friend or acquaintance increases these odds by 2.5 times. Although the level of closeness to the deceased (whether a family member, friend, or acquaintance) does not substantially alter the risk, it is higher when the exposure involves a family member (Hill et al., 2020).

While the mechanisms underlying suicide risk after a loss are not fully understood, depression, along with factors like guilt and stigmatization, are known to play a significant role (Pitman et al., 2014, 2024). Furthermore, exposure to a death by suicide may heighten awareness of suicide as an option and increase knowledge of lethal methods. The increased risk of suicidal behavior among those affected by suicide can also be attributed to prolonged or "complicated grief" (Bellini et al., 2018; Pitman et al., 2014), which is marked by chronicity and intense emotional distress. This condition is associated with persistent intrusive thoughts and memories of the deceased, feelings of guilt and trauma, and significant difficulty in finding meaning in life (Bellini et al., 2018; Mitchell et al., 2004; Pitman et al., 2014).

As a sudden, violent, and unexpected death, often socially sanctioned, that disrupts daily life, grief from suicide presents unique characteristics that distinguish it from other types of grief. Suicide not only generates a feeling of loss; in the early stages of grief, survivors often oscillate between denial of the loss and intrusive thoughts about it. The grief process is often accompanied by feelings of anger or guilt (Why did they do this to me? Could I have prevented it? What did I do wrong?), feelings of abandonment or rejection, shame, and stigmatization (What will others think? How do I explain what happened?), or even thoughts about the meaning of life (What is the purpose of my life now?). Suicide often raises questions that challenge survivors about their role (real or imagined) in the other's death.

Suicide bereavement can be accompanied by various emotions, such as sadness and guilt, but anger is often one of the most reported. This emotion can lead to feelings of shame, as anger and hostility toward someone no longer alive are perceived as inappropriate responses (Causer et al., 2022). Additionally, suicide is often stigmatized, leading survivors to experience shame, feelings of rejection, withdrawal, and social isolation (Pitman et al., 2016). The perceived or internalized stigma associated with suicide adds a burden to the grieving process (Ross et al., 2021).

Socially, the loss from suicide can alter family dynamics, create distancing, and break the usual sources of support for an individual due to the social stigma surrounding suicide. Those grieving a suicide receive less informal support from family and friends compared to those grieving other sudden deaths (McDonnell et al., 2022). Therefore, the reactions of the social and emotional environment can be crucial in shaping the experience and course of the grieving process.

Over a quarter of survivors are estimated to require professional assistance for at least twelve months after the event, and at least a fifth need support for at least two years (McDonnell et al., 2022; Ross et al., 2021). While most individuals grieving a suicide recognize the need for support, they often face numerous barriers that limit their access to care, such as a lack of available services, uncertainty about where to seek help, stigma, and concerns that health services may not view their struggles as serious enough to warrant assistance (Ross et al., 2021). Additionally, both in high-income and middle-income countries, many survivors describe a lack of access to support services due to limitations in the provision of local suicide bereavement support (McDonnell et al., 2022).

It is crucial to recognize that suicide bereavement in childhood and adolescence has distinct characteristics, as young people often express their grief in less apparent ways than adults. In this age group, grief may manifest as anger, guilt, somatic symptoms, avoidance, behavioral changes, insomnia, or physical complaints rather than overt sadness (Bartik et al., 2020; Del Carpio et al., 2021; Pitman et al., 2014). Children and adolescents frequently harbor unspoken questions and concerns about death, underscoring the need for open communication with adults to help them process their emotions and prevent feelings of guilt. Given that adolescence is a stage characterized by emotional turmoil and sensation-seeking, among other aspects, for some adolescents, suicide may appear as a fascinating idea, a potential solution to life's tensions, or a strategy to cope with personal dilemmas (Maples et al., 2005).

To mitigate the detrimental effects of suicide bereavement, access to support services must be timely and available in the long term. International experience suggests the need for "active postvention" that understands the complex nature of suicide bereavement, where support is provided to the affected individuals rather than requiring them to seek out support (Ross et al., 2021). These services should extend their reach to include individuals beyond the immediate family of the deceased, mainly because it is known that those who have lost a friend to suicide suffer mental distress that often goes unaddressed (Feigelman et al., 2018).

10.3 Postvention Strategies

In recent years, postvention has become a focus of international health responses to suicide (Pirkis et al., 2024). The World Health Organization (WHO) has promoted the implementation of postvention interventions, and some national suicide prevention strategies include postvention as a key objective to address the needs of those grieving a suicide (World Health Organization & IASP, 2008).

Currently, various intervention strategies exist to address the impact of a suicide death. Some individual strategies, such as counseling, crisis intervention, or psychotherapy, while others adopt a family or group approach (Bergman et al., 2017; Szumilas & Kutcher, 2011; Maple et al., 2018). There are also community-based strategies, some of which involve peer support groups, while others are led by professionals (Maple et al., 2018).

It is crucial to provide tailored interventions for different groups: individuals directly exposed to the event, vulnerable populations, and the broader community (Séguin et al., 2019). These interventions should be adjusted based on the level of risk, with particular emphasis on those at higher risk of developing medium- and long-term complications (Pirkis et al., 2024). Furthermore, interventions must extend beyond the event's immediate aftermath, with ongoing follow-up to address potential complications or delayed reactions among witnesses, vulnerable groups, and bereaved individuals, lasting at least one year.

Studies have indicated that receiving immediate support after a suicide is associated with a higher likelihood of participating in therapeutic interventions and better psychosocial outcomes, such as reduced loneliness and suicidal ideation (Andriessen et al., 2019a, b; Gehrmann et al., 2020). A recent systematic review examined the acceptability and effectiveness of different types of postvention interventions and found that they can improve the emotional well-being and adjustment of those who have experienced a suicide loss (Abbate et al., 2024). However, knowledge about the various formats and goals of postvention interventions and their feasibility and effectiveness is still limited (Andriessen et al., 2019a, b).

Table 10.1 outlines the various intervention levels aimed at mitigating the effects of suicide exposure.

10.4 Postvention Strategies in the Workplace and Healthcare Services

While most research on suicide bereavement focuses on family members, exposure to suicide in workplace settings has also been documented among police officers, ambulance personnel, mental health professionals, educators, and social care workers (Causer et al., 2022). Despite the professional relationship with the victim, growing evidence indicates that occupational exposure to suicide can result in significant emotional trauma, absenteeism, reduced productivity, and mental health

Table 10.1 Intervention levels to mitigate the impact of suicide exposure

Level of intervention	Description
Universal	This level targets individuals in the general population who may experience emotional distress following indirect exposure to a suicide. Interventions at this stage may include guidelines for responsible communication, as well as information on risk and protective factors associated with suicidal behavior, common psychological reactions, and how to recognize signs of emotional distress in oneself and others. These efforts also aim to reduce stigma around mental health, promote help-seeking behavior, and raise awareness about available support resources.
Selective	This level focuses on individuals who may be at elevated risk due to specific vulnerabilities or circumstances. Interventions include psychoeducational programs and timely information about relevant support services. This level also involves proactively identifying those at higher risk, improving the early detection of mental health problems, and preventing the onset or recurrence of suicidal behavior.
Indicated	This level addresses individuals who have been directly exposed to or affected by a suicide, including those grieving the loss. These individuals may experience intense emotional distress, acute stress, or symptoms of post-traumatic stress disorder. Interventions at this stage focus on providing grief support, alleviating feelings of guilt, and managing suicidal thoughts or behaviors. It is essential that these efforts extend beyond the immediate aftermath to address medium- and long-term emotional and psychological needs.

Source: Jiménez-Molina et al. (2025)
Note: Individuals who require indicated-level interventions may also benefit from universal and selective interventions

issues (Aldrich & Cerel, 2022; Kinman & Torry, 2021; Lyra et al., 2021; Nelson et al., 2020).

The impact of losing a colleague to suicide in the workplace presents significant challenges as organizations struggle to balance their operational needs with providing adequate support to affected individuals (Causer et al., 2022). A lack of time and emotional support often exacerbates this difficulty, leading employees to feel abandoned and silenced, even when there is a strong need to discuss the event openly (Causer et al., 2022; Kinman & Torry, 2021). The pressure to return to "normal" and the emphasis on "moving on" can obscure the emotional distress some staff may be experiencing, creating a disconnect between organizational expectations and individual needs (Causer et al., 2022; Kinman & Torry, 2021). This tension is further complicated by the organization's unpreparedness to address suicide loss, which can perpetuate feelings of stigma and hinder the grieving process by making employees feel their needs are unacknowledged (Causer et al., 2022).

The experiences of workers' loss and grief due to suicide are influenced by workplace characteristics, the nature of roles, and professional identities (Causer et al., 2022). Certain workplace cultures can affect whether workers feel comfortable expressing emotions or seeking help. For instance, exposure to patient suicide is a common occupational risk for mental health and social work professionals (Leaune et al., 2019; Séguin et al., 2014). It is estimated that about one-third of social workers (Jacobson et al., 2004), 55% of nurses (Takahashi et al., 2011), between 22% and 39% of psychologists (Castelli et al., 2017), and between 51% and 82% of psychiatrists (Castelli et al., 2017) will be exposed to a patient's suicide at some point in their careers. Some professionals may positively manage the impact of suicide, viewing it as a learning experience. However, others may experience emotional effects that affect their performance and make them feel like failures or powerless for not fulfilling their duty of care, or even frustrated because their efforts to help seem futile (Leaune et al., 2020). For some healthcare professionals, this can lead to experiencing "disenfranchised grief," grief denied recognition because society and colleagues do not consider their impact legitimate since they are not family members or loved ones of the deceased (Leaune et al., 2020). Moreover, the dual roles that healthcare professionals must assume, providing support to others while grieving themselves, add a layer of complexity. This can undermine self-confidence and professional competence, leading to avoidance of patients with suicidal risk and a decrease in effective decision-making.

Despite growing evidence on the impact of workplace suicide exposure, especially among healthcare professionals, the lack of institutional support has been widely documented (Castelli et al., 2017; Causer et al., 2022; Leaune et al., 2019). Although some postvention guidelines exist to help workers affected by a colleague's suicide (Kinman & Torry, 2021), the existing evidence is limited.

Retrospective studies have revealed that support from peers, supervisors, or the institution can be both a protective factor and a predictor of adaptive coping strategies and lower levels of emotional impact and trauma (Castelli et al., 2017). For example, in France, the effectiveness of the SUPPORT program, which provides support to healthcare professionals exposed to a patient's suicide, is currently being evaluated (Leaune et al., 2020). In the United Kingdom, the PABBS program trained healthcare professionals in supporting parents who have lost a child to suicide (McDonnell et al., 2020). The pilot evaluation significantly improved professionals' knowledge, skills, and confidence. A study on a mutual support group for psychiatrists dealing with patient suicides indicates that professional peer participation is beneficial for the grieving process (Tamworth et al., 2022).

These experiences suggest that providing time and emotional space for processing and grieving in the workplace can be beneficial in addressing the emotional labor that may arise after a loss in workplace settings. They also suggest that postvention strategies must be sensitive to the specific needs of professional groups and cultures.

10.5 Postvention Strategies in Educational Settings

Suicide in the school context is an event that affects the entire educational community, including children, adolescents, teachers, and administrative staff. A study on the immediate impact of a student's suicide revealed that over 67% of teachers experienced personal and professional effects (Kõlves et al., 2017). Teachers expressed significant distress when supporting at-risk students, with nearly a third reporting a loss of confidence in handling such situations. While 65% turned to family and partners for support, 27% highlighted the need for specific resources, including counseling, crisis management training, and professional assistance. Many teachers feel unprepared to support grieving students and struggle to access appropriate mental health resources.

A similar situation is observed in higher education institutions. Despite suicide being the second leading cause of death among young people, universities often lack the necessary tools to address and respond to student suicide emergencies (Allie et al., 2023). University staff frequently feel that the institution's response focuses more on student well-being and does not adequately address their needs (Allie et al., 2023). Student affairs administrators often lack the necessary preparation to effectively address suicide on campus and highlight key concerns such as the lack of training in suicide prevention and postvention, difficulties in communicating and officially notifying the suicide—particularly in balancing privacy with timely information dissemination and responsible handling on social media. Additionally, they face the challenge of balancing the commemoration of the student's death with the risk of social contagion of suicidal behaviors. Another key challenge is the lack of evaluated postvention interventions in universities. A systematic review found that no studies directly address such interventions in these institutions (Allie et al., 2023).

The literature identifies several key postvention strategies in educational settings. One practical approach is the creation of a community response plan, where teachers, mental health professionals, and crisis support teams collaborate to identify and refer high-risk individuals to mental health services (Andriessen et al., 2019a, b; Cox et al., 2012; Szumilas & Kutcher, 2011). Another strategy involves psychoeducational workshops, which raise awareness of suicide warning signs and equip community members with crisis-coping strategies to encourage early intervention and connection to psychological support (Andriessen et al., 2019a, b).

In addition, individual or group counseling is recommended for those grappling with complex emotions following a suicide, addressing grief, challenges in interpreting suicidal behavior, and facilitating access to appropriate services. Screening for at-risk students, particularly after a community suicide, has also proven effective in identifying high-risk individuals and increasing their likelihood of receiving mental health support. Training teachers and staff to recognize and assist at-risk students plays a critical role in all these interventions (Cox et al., 2012).

Although various postvention strategies in the school context are described in the literature, their evaluation is limited, and results vary significantly. For example, a study in Korea reported positive outcomes in reducing psychological distress and traumatic symptoms after implementing a crisis intervention one week following a student's suicide (Cha et al., 2018). In contrast, another study involving students selected by school staff for their closeness to the deceased found no significant effects on depression, risk behaviors, suicidal ideation, or alcohol and drug use (Hazell & Lewin, 1993). A recent study evaluated the effectiveness of an online role-playing simulation aimed at training educators and school staff to manage death and suicide in educational settings (Khalid et al., 2022). The program was found to improve participants' ability to recognize signs of psychological distress, enhance their preparedness and confidence in discussing support services with students and colleagues, and reduce the stigma surrounding mental health and suicide.

Most information on postvention in educational settings is presented as technical guidelines for implementing community-based interventions (Andriessen et al., 2019a, b; Maples et al., 2005). These guidelines primarily focus on immediate responses following a suicide, but some also stress the importance of ongoing support, supervision, and careful management of information, including on social media (Cox et al., 2016; Maples et al., 2005; Marshall et al., 2018). A key element in these guides is the establishment of a Crisis Response Team to oversee and implement intervention strategies (Andriessen et al., 2019a, b; Cox et al., 2016; Maples et al., 2005). Teachers are particularly well-positioned to contribute to prevention efforts by recognizing early warning signs of mental health issues in students (Kõlves et al., 2017). Additionally, postvention guidelines recommend funeral rituals, commemoration, and the return to routine. While these rituals and events are important for processing the loss and fostering community cohesion, finding a balance between providing space for commemoration and avoiding the idealization of the deceased remains a significant challenge.

Table 10.2 presents the key dimensions for addressing a suicide crisis in educational settings.

Table 10.2 Key dimensions for responding to a suicide crisis in educational settings

Moment	Description
Prior to the crisis	*Establish a crisis response team*: The crisis response team comprises various professionals, including administrators, counselors, social workers, psychologists, nurses, and an ICT expert to handle social media. The team must be skilled in collaborating with all groups within the school community.
Crisis: Shock and disorganization	*Initial reactions and immediate response*: At this stage, reactions of shock and denial typically arise. The response team should be activated to manage the suspected suicidal behavior and act as a liaison with the deceased student's family. Additionally, they are responsible for informing school staff, students, parents, and the broader community about the suicide. *Communication and support*: It is essential to approach students and the broader community with empathy, active listening, and avoiding judgment. Key steps include managing the deceased student's belongings and providing psychological first aid to those affected. *Regulation of daily functional rhythms*: Concrete responses to regulate daily routines, such as managing sleep, anxiety, and insomnia, are important. These strategies may include relaxation techniques to improve concentration and overall well-being. *Media and social media management*: Handling the media and managing the Internet and social media must be done carefully and strategically to prevent the spread of erroneous or harmful information. *Access to support services*: Information on how to access support services should be included to ensure everyone has the resources they need during this difficult time.

(continued)

Table 10.2 (continued)

Moment	Description
Crisis: Expression of emotions	*Facilitation of emotional expression*: Trained personnel should recognize that heightened emotions can intensify grief and trigger crises, often leading to feelings of guilt, with thoughts like "if only I had reacted differently." Facilitating funeral rituals is crucial to encourage emotional expression and foster group solidarity during this process. *Psychological first aid*: Psychological first aid aims to help individuals make sense of the event, teach coping techniques for managing negative thoughts, and acknowledge the permanence of the loss. *Support for high-risk students*: Identifying high-risk students and providing ongoing support is essential. Counselors play a key role in dispelling rumors, sharing accurate information, and normalizing grief reactions, highlighting that these responses are individual and expected. This can be facilitated by distributing brochures and other educational materials to the community. *Support for school staff*: Ongoing support for school staff is vital to ensure an environment of mutual support and emotional well-being.
Exploring the significance of the loss	*Grief and reintegration*: At this stage, as the initial intensity of grief subsides and daily routines resume, students often enter a phase of questioning. They seek new ways to understand their reality and restore meaning and purpose in their lives after the disruption caused by the loss. *Continuous support and counseling*: Continuous, scheduled counseling is essential at multiple levels. For students, both individual and group support helps them process their emotions. The parent community should receive ongoing guidance and resources to support their children better. At the same time, school staff need consistent emotional support to foster a supportive environment and ensure their well-being. *Mental health education*: Educate about the differences between adaptive emotional reactions (sadness) and mental health issues (depression). The focus should be on encouraging timely help-seeking and teaching how to recognize signs and symptoms, ensuring that students and staff receive the appropriate support when needed.
Development of new understandings and goals, and return to a (new) daily life	*New understandings and planning*: This phase is marked by gaining new insights and making plans. It also allows the team to evaluate their efforts, identifying key issues and areas for improvement. *Continuous monitoring*: Constant monitoring of both students and staff is crucial to ensure their well-being. Maintaining detailed records and documentation helps refine support practices and strategies for ongoing improvement. *Self-care*: Promote self-care and regularly evaluate the team to ensure their well-being and effectiveness in their roles.

Note: Adapted from Cox et al. (2016) and Maples et al. (2005)

10.6 Psychotherapy and Psychoeducational Approaches

Psychotherapeutic interventions for suicide survivors primarily focus on helping individuals process their emotions and adjust to their new life without necessarily seeking to break the bond with the deceased. Existing literature highlights various available support strategies, including crisis intervention, psychotherapy, counseling, and psychoeducational approaches. These strategies can be implemented individually, in groups, or through both modalities.

Crisis intervention is often the first psychotherapeutic contact with survivors, focusing on providing emotional containment, psychoeducation, counseling, and a psychological assessment (Cha et al., 2018; Poijula et al., 2001). This intervention is suitable for various settings, including schools and workplaces, and is most effective in the early stages of grief. An example is the "StandBy Response Service" program, which offers in-person or telephone support by a crisis response team. Studies indicate that this service reduces self-reported suicidal tendencies and improves users' quality of life and psychological health (Visser et al., 2014).

Psychoeducational interventions play a crucial role in grief management by creating spaces for survivors to express their emotions while providing specific information and counseling about suicide grief. These interventions blend counseling and psychotherapy, encouraging survivors to confront their loss, address grief symptoms, and develop coping skills. For example, an 8-session group program led by a psychologist and a trained survivor volunteer improved emotional regulation and reduced grief-related symptoms (Farberow, 1992). Home visits by clinical psychologists effectively addressed depression, complicated grief, and suicide risk by correcting misconceptions about suicide and promoting healthy coping strategies (Wittouck et al., 2014). Similarly, counseling and cognitive-behavioral training provided by psychiatric nursing staff aimed to prevent complicated grief among surviving family members, with a 12-month follow-up showing fewer maladaptive grief reactions and feelings of guilt (de Groot et al., 2007).

For children and adolescents, tailored psychoeducational interventions have yielded promising outcomes. A 10-week group intervention significantly reduced anxiety and depressive symptoms in young participants (Pfeffer et al., 2002). The online program "Let's Talk Suicide" helps children cope with grief after losing a parent or sibling, fostering connections between guardians and providing opportunities for the bereaved to support others (Krysinska et al., 2024). Additionally, the "Waves" program, offering therapeutic support through narrative techniques and autobiographical storytelling for parents and children, has been highly rated for its blend of professional guidance and personal experience (Bowden, 2011).

Psychotherapeutic interventions for suicide survivors typically focus on addressing complicated grief, with cognitive-behavioral techniques being central to treating avoidant behaviors related to grief-associated thoughts and feelings (Neimeyer, 2000; Shear et al., 2005). Key clinical tasks include containing trauma, restoring emotional regulation, creating new personal narratives, developing social skills, and reconciling the bond with the deceased (Jordan & McGann, 2017).

Cognitive-behavioral therapy (CBT) conceptualizes complicated grief as resulting from three interrelated processes: insufficient integration of the loss into autobiographical memory, negative beliefs and catastrophic interpretations about grief, and the use of anxious or depressive avoidance strategies (Boelen, 2006). CBT interventions focus on psychoeducation about complicated grief and use techniques such as exposure to grief cues, cognitive restructuring, and behavioral activation. The primary goal is to foster adaptive responses, enabling individuals to share their experiences and enhance self-observation and self-regulation skills.

Many psychotherapeutic approaches are based on models such as the Dual Process Model of Grief (Stroebe & Schut, 1999), which contrasts with traditional stage theories by proposing that grief oscillates between two key dimensions: loss and restoration. The loss dimension involves processing the emotional impact of the loss, while the restoration dimension centers on adapting to life without the deceased. Effective integration of these processes is essential for adapting to the loss while maintaining a continuing bond with the deceased.

For instance, complicated grief therapy (CGT) is based on the premise that acute grief can be transformed into integrated grief by addressing the complications in the grief process (Shear & Shair, 2005). CGT is available in various formats, including internet-supported (Tur et al., 2022) and group settings (Supiano et al., 2017), blending motivational interviewing, CBT, and prolonged exposure therapy elements.

Despite the variety of therapeutic approaches, the literature shows mixed results regarding their effectiveness (Andriessen et al. 2019a, b; Linde et al., 2017; Mcdaid et al., 2008; Szumilas & Kutcher, 2011). Several factors contribute to this inconsistency, including the heterogeneity of outcome measures and methodological variability across studies (de Groot et al., 2007; Supiano et al., 2017; Wittouck et al., 2014; Zisook et al., 2018). Nonetheless, psychotherapeutic interventions remain essential in supporting survivors, particularly in alleviating grief-related symptoms. For instance, interventions based on CBT and CGT have been effective in reducing symptoms such as intrusive thoughts, social isolation, and maladaptive avoidance behaviors (Boelen, 2006; Supiano et al., 2017; Tur et al., 2022; Zisook et al., 2018). Despite their limitations, these interventions significantly contribute to the emotional recovery of survivors.

10.7 Alternative Therapeutic Strategies

Alternative therapeutic strategies for suicide survivors focus on creating narratives around the loss and regaining a sense of control over their lives. Writing exercises, for example, have been shown to reduce the pain and intensity of grief related to suicide (Kovac & Range, 2000). Weekend retreats for survivors, which combine mindfulness with therapeutic techniques, promote acceptance, forgiveness, and anger management (Scocco et al., 2019).

Interventions in natural settings, such as grief camps, provide short-term support for grieving children and adolescents, guided by professionals and volunteers (Clute

& Kobayashi, 2013). These camps, informed by approaches like family therapy and trauma-focused CBT, offer a psychoeducational space where participants can discuss their loss, engage in social activities, and learn healthy coping strategies through games and sports. By fostering connections with others who share similar experiences, both retreats and grief camps help reduce feelings of guilt, shame, and stigma associated with grief from suicide.

Research shows that grief camps are effective, with participants demonstrating improved coping skills, reduced anxiety, enhanced self-esteem, decreased shame and guilt, and better family communication (Hartwig & Marlow, 2022).

10.8 Suicide Bereavement Support Groups

In recent decades, mutual support groups have emerged as a prominent mental health intervention grounded in community-based initiatives emphasizing mutual assistance, self-determination, and agency (Solomon, 2004). These groups bring together individuals facing similar challenges, such as illness, loss, or life experiences (Calcaterra & Raineri, 2020), with specific groups designed for survivors of suicide loss. A recent systematic review found that these groups primarily consist of adults, especially parents, with many female participants (Inostroza et al., 2023). The groups are typically facilitated by peer experts, mental health professionals, or a combination.

The core idea is that sharing information, emotions, and experiences in a safe space fosters connection and support among participants (Ali & Lucock, 2020; Groos & Shakespeare-Finch, 2013). Survivors join these groups to connect with others who have faced similar losses, helping them better understand their grief and form a collective identity as "survivors," which fosters a sense of belonging (Higgins et al., 2022). This connection plays a crucial role in reducing feelings of guilt, isolation, and stigma often linked to suicide-related grief (Ali & Lucock, 2020; Groos & Shakespeare-Finch, 2013; Hybholt et al., 2022; Testoni et al., 2019).

These groups offer a stigma-free environment where participants can share coping strategies, acknowledging the individuality of the grieving process (Hybholt et al., 2022; Supiano, 2012). A key motivation for participants is the search for meaning in the aftermath of suicide, achieved by sharing experiences and knowledge with other survivors. This process helps them construct new narratives around the death, facilitating meaning-making, which is essential for understanding the impact of the loss and maintaining "continuing bonds" with the deceased (Ali & Lucock, 2020; Goodall et al., 2022; Higgins et al., 2022).

Peer support services for survivors are available in both in-person and online formats (Inostroza et al., 2023). Comparative studies have shown mixed results: one study found that online participants experienced higher levels of distress than those in in-person groups. However, they felt their needs were better met online (Feigelman et al., 2008). Conversely, other studies concluded that online support was as beneficial as in-person support (Inostroza et al., 2023).

While mutual support groups hold promise in reducing self-blame, isolation, and stigma during the grieving process, further research is needed to understand group dynamics, participant retention, and the overall effectiveness of these groups (Andriessen et al., 2019a, b; Ali & Lucock, 2020; Higgins et al., 2022; Hybholt et al., 2022). A study from Denmark and Ireland identified three key characteristics of survivor support groups (Hybholt et al., 2022). First, they function as "transformative spaces," offering new perspectives that aid the grieving process. Second, they provide "alternative spaces for belonging and grieving" where individuals can express their emotions without judgment. Lastly, they are described as "conflict spaces," where participants find comfort but struggle with the paradoxical desire not to belong to them.

In addition to mutual aid groups, specialized programs like the Survivors of Suicide Attempts (SOSA) support program in the United States offer targeted support for those who have survived a suicide attempt (Hom et al., 2018). The SOSA program consists of eight closed group sessions led by a professional facilitator and a peer expert. Evaluations have demonstrated positive outcomes, including high adherence and engagement, along with significant reductions in suicidal ideation and attempts.

The WHO (2021) has recommended integrating support groups for suicide loss survivors into national suicide prevention strategies, a practice increasingly adopted in Europe, the United States, and Australia since 2000 (Inostroza et al., 2023). These mutual support groups, implemented mainly by non-governmental organizations in high-income countries (Higgins et al., 2022), are crucial in supporting survivors. However, despite some guidelines from organizations like the WHO and IASP (World Health Organization & IASP, 2008), there remains a lack of technical guidance for establishing and effectively running these groups. This gap extends to the role of local health teams in promoting and supporting these groups within health centers and integrating them into national suicide prevention programs.

The groups need to be linked to the health system and supervised by professional facilitators to monitor potential risks, but clear, comprehensive guidelines are still lacking. While international guidelines on peer support groups exist (National Action Alliance for Suicide Prevention: Suicide Attempt Survivors Task Force, 2014), evidence on the effectiveness of mutual aid groups remains limited (Cook et al., 2017; Higgins et al., 2022; Inostroza et al., 2023; Schlichthorst et al., 2020).

Evaluating the effectiveness of peer or mutual aid support groups is challenging due to the lack of a clear definition and the absence of control groups in most studies, making it difficult to attribute observed effects solely to group participation (Ali & Lucock, 2020; Groos & Shakespeare-Finch, 2013). Additionally, the diversity within groups—such as differences between losing a child versus a partner—can reduce the sense of community, highlighting the need for more homogeneous group compositions.

Open groups face additional issues, such as discomfort among long-term members due to the frequent introduction of new participants, which can also create barriers for newcomers (Inostroza et al., 2023; Testoni et al., 2019). Moreover, participation in these groups can sometimes lead to distress or depression, with sessions potentially triggering negative thoughts (Higgins et al., 2022; Hybholt et al.,

2022). In the case of peer support among families of military suicide survivors in the U.S., risks like re-victimization or feeling overwhelmed by others' pain have been reported, indicating that these groups may not be suitable for everyone (Harrington-LaMorie et al., 2018).

10.9 What Should We Know?

Over the past two decades, research on suicide bereavement has grown substantially, making postvention a key focus in international health responses (Abbate et al., 2024; Gehrmann et al., 2020; Pirkis et al., 2024). Both research and clinical practice have highlighted that suicide survivors are at high risk of developing mental health issues and suicidal behaviors, often exacerbated by inadequate guidance from healthcare providers. This underscores the need for a proactive postvention approach, where health professionals and institutions across workplace, educational, and healthcare settings are trained to recognize and address grief and manage mental health warning signs.

Several postvention strategies have been developed to support suicide survivors. These interventions should be customized for specific target groups (directly exposed individuals, vulnerable populations, and the broader community) and adapted to the appropriate level of risk. Psychotherapeutic interventions aid in emotional processing, grief management, and adapting to a new reality. Mutual support groups have also proven to be essential, providing a space to alleviate feelings of guilt, isolation, and stigma. Intensive support, which combines therapeutic and educational components, offers immediate assistance and ongoing followup. While some studies indicate that these supports are perceived as effective in reducing depressive symptoms and uncomplicated grief, their impact on lowering suicide risk remains uncertain (Andriessen et al., 2019a, b; Hill et al., 2020). This suggests that more targeted interventions may be necessary, with trained professionals equipped to address both the loss from suicide and active suicidal thoughts and behaviors.

CBT is the predominant therapeutic approach in postvention, while interventions based on psychodynamic approaches are less common. Although suicide research primarily focuses on the individual, it is crucial to consider contextual and organizational factors for a more comprehensive understanding of grief and more effective interventions. Group interventions remain the most common form of postvention, although they tend to attract more women and underrepresent children, adolescents, and older adults (Andriessen et al., 2019a, b). Despite the low quality of many studies, evidence supports their effectiveness in the grief process. However, challenges remain, such as maintaining a sense of group, integrating new participants, and providing adequate support.

The use of digital technologies in postvention is an emerging area that requires further exploration. Online resources offer an effective alternative for improving early access to help and reducing barriers such as shame, stigma, cost, and geographical distance (Krysinska & Andriessen, 2017; Lestienne et al., 2021). However, little is known about the needs and expectations of bereaved individuals regarding digital resources. A study found that three-quarters of suicide survivors used the Internet during their grief, primarily to obtain information on suicide bereavement and prevention, as well as to access testimonies from others in similar situations (Leaune et al., 2022). These findings highlight the need to develop digital interventions that provide reliable information and professional support and innovate by integrating both in-person and remote components, going beyond simply replicating traditional methods.

Despite the growth of postvention research over the past decade (Maple et al., 2018), global evidence remains limited (Andriessen et al., 2019a, b; Inostroza et al., 2023). Significant knowledge gaps persist, highlighting the need for continued research and improvements in clinical practice to support suicide survivors better.

One of the significant challenges in suicide bereavement research is the lack of studies conducted in diverse contexts, particularly in regions like Latin America, where there is a significant research gap. Most studies (93%) are concentrated in high-income countries in the Global North (Allie et al., 2023), leading to a geographic bias that restricts a comprehensive global understanding of suicide bereavement. To correct this imbalance, expanding research efforts and incorporating a broader range of cultural and contextual perspectives is essential.

Generating robust evidence in postvention research presents significant challenges, particularly in diversifying samples by age and gender. Studies often overrepresent women and underrepresent older adults, despite older adults and men accounting for most suicides in many countries (Bennett et al., 2023). Further research is needed to explore how cultural norms of masculinity and other barriers affect help-seeking behavior and suicide risk among male survivors. Moreover, future research should prioritize children and adolescents who are often overlooked.

A key challenge in suicide research is the limited inclusion of perspectives from survivors and individuals with lived experience. Their involvement in prevention and postvention programs has proven valuable for developing peer support initiatives and introducing innovative approaches. Studies show that integrating lived experience into prevention strategies offers significant benefits, such as enhancing feelings of being heard and improving crisis management skills (Watling et al., 2022).

Despite mental health policies promoting the inclusion of these voices for over three decades, a significant gap remains in their full integration (Lezine, 2016; Watling et al., 2022). As this practice is still relatively recent, it is crucial to establish clear guidelines for effectively incorporating it into postvention strategies. Many survivor inclusion initiatives have yet to be fully explored, underscoring the need to eliminate barriers that impede active participation. The development of future services must be guided by the insights of those affected by suicide, ensuring that interventions are tailored to meet their needs.

Acknowledgments This manuscript was supported by ANID—Millennium Science Initiative Program—AIM23_0002 and NCS2021_081 and by ANID—FONIS SA23I0181. We express our gratitude to Paulina del Río for her valuable contribution to the development of the postvention field in Chile.

References

Abbate, L., Chopra, J., Poole, H., & Saini, P. (2024). Evaluating postvention services and the acceptability of models of postvention: A systematic review. *Omega, 90*(2), 865–905. https://doi.org/10.1177/00302228221112723

Aldrich, R. S., & Cerel, J. (2022). Occupational suicide exposure and impact on Mental Health: Examining differences across helping professions. *Omega, 85*(1), 23–37. https://doi.org/10.1177/0030222820933019

Ali, F., & Lucock, M. (2020). 'It's like getting a group hug and you can cry there and be yourself and they understand'. Family members' experiences of using a suicide bereavement peer support group. *Bereavement Care, 39*(2), 51–58. https://doi.org/10.1080/02682621.2020.1771951

Allie, S. N., Bantjes, J., & Andriessen, K. (2023). Suicide postvention for staff and students on university campuses: A scoping review. *BMJ Open, 13*(6), e068730. https://doi.org/10.1136/bmjopen-2022-068730

Andriessen, K., Rahman, B., Draper, B., Dudley, M., & Mitchell, P. B. (2017). Prevalence of exposure to suicide: A meta-analysis of population-based studies. *Journal of Psychiatric Research, 88*, 113–120. https://doi.org/10.1016/j.jpsychires.2017.01.017

Andriessen, K., Krysinska, K., Hill, N. T. M., Reifels, L., Robinson, J., Reavley, N., & Pirkis, J. (2019a). Effectiveness of interventions for people bereaved through suicide: A systematic review of controlled studies of grief, psychosocial and suicide-related outcomes. *BMC Psychiatry, 19*(1), 49. https://doi.org/10.1186/s12888-019-2020-z

Andriessen, K., Krysinska, K., Kõlves, K., & Reavley, N. (2019b). Suicide postvention service models and guidelines 2014–2019: A systematic review. *Frontiers in Psychology, 10*, 2677. https://doi.org/10.3389/fpsyg.2019.02677

Bartik, W. J., Maple, M., & McKay, K. (2020). Youth suicide bereavement and the continuum of risk. *Crisis, 41*(6), 483–489. https://doi.org/10.1027/0227-5910/a000653

Bellini, S., Erbuto, D., Andriessen, K., Milelli, M., Innamorati, M., Lester, D., Sampogna, G., Fiorillo, A., & Pompili, M. (2018). Depression, hopelessness, and complicated grief in survivors of suicide. *Frontiers in Psychology, 9*, 198. https://doi.org/10.3389/fpsyg.2018.00198

Bennett, S., Robb, K. A., Zortea, T. C., Dickson, A., Richardson, C., & O'Connor, R. C. (2023). Male suicide risk and recovery factors: A systematic review and qualitative metasynthesis of two decades of research. *Psychological Bulletin, 149*(7–8), 371–417. https://doi.org/10.1037/bul0000397

Bergman, A. S., Axberg, U., & Hanson, E. (2017). When a parent dies – A systematic review of the effects of support programs for parentally bereaved children and their caregivers. *BMC Palliative Care, 16*(1), 39. https://doi.org/10.1186/s12904-017-0223-y

Boelen, P. A. (2006). Cognitive-behavioral therapy for complicated grief: Theoretical underpinnings and case descriptions. *Journal of Loss and Trauma, 11*(1), 1–30. https://doi.org/10.1080/15325020500193655

Bowden, C. (2011). Waves: A psycho-educational programme for adults bereaved by suicide. *Bereavement Care, 30*(3), 25–31. https://doi.org/10.1080/02682621.2011.617970

Calcaterra, V., & Raineri, M. L. (2020). Helping each other: A peer supervision group with facilitators of mutual aid groups. *Social Work With Groups, 43*(4), 351–364. https://doi.org/10.1080/01609513.2019.1642829

Castelli, D., Treven, M., Grad, O. T., & Andriessen, K. (2017). Impact of client suicide on health and mental health professionals. In K. Andriessen, K. Krysinska, & O. T. Grad (Eds.), *Postvention in action: The international handbook of suicide bereavement support* (pp. 245–254). Hogrefe Publishing.

Causer, H., Spiers, J., Efstathiou, N., Aston, S., Chew-Graham, C. A., Gopfert, A., Grayling, K., Maben, J., van Hove, M., & Riley, R. (2022). The impact of colleague suicide and the current state of postvention guidance for affected co-workers: A critical integrative review. *International Journal of Environmental Research and Public Health, 19*(18), 11565. https://doi.org/10.3390/ijerph191811565

Cerel, J., McIntosh, J. L., Neimeyer, R. A., Maple, M., & Marshall, D. (2014). The continuum of "survivorship": Definitional issues in the aftermath of suicide. *Suicide & Life-Threatening Behavior, 44*(6), 591–600. https://doi.org/10.1111/sltb.12093

Cerel, J., Brown, M. M., Maple, M., Singleton, M., van de Venne, J., Moore, M., & Flaherty, C. (2019). How many people are exposed to suicide? Not Six. *Suicide & Life-threatening Behavior, 49*(2), 529–534. https://doi.org/10.1111/sltb.12450

Cha, J. M., Kim, J. E., Kim, M. A., Shim, B., Cha, M. J., Lee, J. J., Han, D. H., & Chung, U. S. (2018). Five months follow-up study of school-based crisis intervention for Korean High School students who experienced a peer suicide. *Journal of Korean Medical Science, 33*(28), e192. https://doi.org/10.3346/jkms.2018.33.e192

Clute, M. A., & Kobayashi, R. (2013). Are children's grief camps effective? *Journal of Social Work in End-of-Life & Palliative Care, 9*(1), 43–57. https://doi.org/10.1080/15524256.2013.758927

Cook, F. J., Langford, L., & Ruocco, K. (2017). Evidence- and practice-informed approach to implementing peer grief support after suicide systematically in the USA. *Death Studies, 41*(10), 648–658. https://doi.org/10.1080/07481187.2017.1335552

Cox, G. R., Robinson, J., Williamson, M., Lockley, A., Cheung, Y. T., & Pirkis, J. (2012). Suicide clusters in young people: Evidence for the effectiveness of postvention strategies. *Crisis, 33*(4), 208–214. https://doi.org/10.1027/0227-5910/a000144

Cox, G. R., Bailey, E., Jorm, A. F., Reavley, N. J., Templer, K., Parker, A., Rickwood, D., Bhar, S., & Robinson, J. (2016). Development of suicide postvention guidelines for secondary schools: A Delphi study. *BMC Public Health, 16*, 180. https://doi.org/10.1186/s12889-016-2822-6

Del Carpio, L., Paul, S., Paterson, A., & Rasmussen, S. (2021). A systematic review of controlled studies of suicidal and self-harming behaviours in adolescents following bereavement by suicide. *PLoS One, 16*(7), e0254203. https://doi.org/10.1371/journal.pone.0254203

Farberow, N. L. (1992). The Los Angeles Survivors-After-Suicide program. An evaluation. *Crisis, 13*(1), 23–34.

Feigelman, W., Gorman, B. S., Beal, K. C., & Jordan, J. R. (2008). Internet support groups for suicide survivors: A new mode for gaining bereavement assistance. *Omega, 57*(3), 217–243. https://doi.org/10.2190/OM.57.3.a

Feigelman, W., Cerel, J., McIntosh, J. L., Brent, D., & Gutin, N. (2018). Suicide exposures and bereavement among American adults: Evidence from the 2016 General Social Survey. *Journal of Affective Disorders, 227*, 1–6. https://doi.org/10.1016/j.jad.2017.09.056

Gehrmann, M., Dixon, S. D., Visser, V. S., & Griffin, M. (2020). Evaluating the outcomes for bereaved people supported by a community-based suicide bereavement service. *Crisis, 41*(6), 437–444. https://doi.org/10.1027/0227-5910/a000658

Goodall, R., Krysinska, K., & Andriessen, K. (2022). Continuing bonds after loss by suicide: A systematic review. *International Journal of Environmental Research and Public Health, 19*(5), 2963. https://doi.org/10.3390/ijerph19052963

Groos, A. D., & Shakespeare-Finch, J. (2013). Positive experiences for participants in suicide bereavement groups: A grounded theory model. *Death Studies, 37*(1), 1–24. https://doi.org/10.1080/07481187.2012.687898

de Groot, M., & Kollen, B. J. (2013). Course of bereavement over 8–10 years in first degree relatives and spouses of people who committed suicide: Longitudinal community based cohort study. *BMJ (Clinical research ed.), 347*, f5519. https://doi.org/10.1136/bmj.f5519

de Groot, M., de Keijser, J., Neeleman, J., Kerkhof, A., Nolen, W., & Burger, H. (2007). Cognitive behaviour therapy to prevent complicated grief among relatives and spouses bereaved by suicide: Cluster randomised controlled trial. *BMJ (Clinical research ed.), 334*(7601), 994. https://doi.org/10.1136/bmj.39161.457431.55

Harrington-LaMorie, J., Jordan, J. R., Ruocco, K., & Cerel, J. (2018). Surviving families of military suicide loss: Exploring postvention peer support. *Death Studies, 42*(3), 143–154. https://doi.org/10.1080/07481187.2017.1370789

Hartwig, E. K., & Marlow, M. (2022). Finding hope at camp: An investigation of the influence of grief camp on youth depression, anxiety, and self-concept indicators. *Journal of Loss and Trauma, 27*(2), 149–158. https://doi.org/10.1080/15325024.2021.1913926

Hazell, P., & Lewin, T. (1993). An evaluation of postvention following adolescent suicide. *Suicide & Life-Threatening Behavior, 23*(2), 101–109. https://doi.org/10.1111/j.1943-278X.1993.tb00374.x

Higgins, A., Hybholt, L., Meuser, O. A., Eustace Cook, J., Downes, C., & Morrissey, J. (2022). Scoping review of peer-led support for people bereaved by suicide. *International Journal of Environmental Research and Public Health, 19*(6), 3485. https://doi.org/10.3390/ijerph19063485

Hill, N. T. M., Robinson, J., Pirkis, J., Andriessen, K., Krysinska, K., Payne, A., Boland, A., Clarke, A., Milner, A., Witt, K., Krohn, S., & Lampit, A. (2020). Association of suicidal behavior with exposure to suicide and suicide attempt: A systematic review and multilevel meta-analysis. *PLoS Medicine, 17*(3), e1003074. https://doi.org/10.1371/journal.pmed.1003074

Hom, M. A., Davis, L., & Joiner, T. E. (2018). Survivors of suicide attempts (SOSA) support group: Preliminary findings from an open-label trial. *Psychological Services, 15*(3), 289–297. https://doi.org/10.1037/ser0000195

Hybholt, L., Higgins, A., Buus, N., Berring, L. L., Connolly, T., Erlangsen, A., & Morrissey, J. (2022). The spaces of peer-led support groups for suicide bereaved in Denmark and the Republic of Ireland: A Focus Group Study. *International Journal of Environmental Research and Public Health, 19*(16), 9898. https://doi.org/10.3390/ijerph19169898

Inostroza, C., Rubio-Ramirez, F., Bustos, C., Quijada, Y., Fernández, D., Bühring, V., et al. (2023). Peer-support groups for suicide loss survivors: A systematic review. *Social Work With Groups, 47*(3), 234–250. https://doi.org/10.1080/01609513.2023.2249053

Jacobson, J. M., Ting, L., Sanders, S., & Harrington, D. (2004). Prevalence of and reactions to fatal and nonfatal client suicidal behavior: A national study of mental health social workers. *Omega: Journal of Death and Dying, 49*(3), 237–248. https://doi.org/10.2190/HPKQ-T700-EPQL-58JQ

Jiménez-Molina, A., Costa-Cordella, S., Rojas, G., Martínez, V., del Río, P., Silva, M., Barrera, T., Ojeda, F., & Núñez, D. (2025). *Estar: Guía de postvención para el acompañamiento de personas, familias y comunidades tras una muerte por suicidio*. Santiago, Chile.

Jordan, J. R., & McGann, V. (2017). Clinical work with suicide loss survivors: Implications of the U.S. postvention guidelines. *Death Studies, 41*(10), 659–672. https://doi.org/10.1080/07481187.2017.1335553

Khalid, N., Zapparrata, N., Loughlin, K., & Albright, G. (2022). Postvention as prevention: Coping with loss at school. *International Journal of Environmental Research and Public Health, 19*(18), 11795. https://doi.org/10.3390/ijerph191811795

Kinman, G., & Torry, R. (2021). Developing a suicide postvention framework for staff in primary healthcare. *Occupational Medicine (Oxford, England), 71*(4–5), 171–173. https://doi.org/10.1093/occmed/kqaa192

Kõlves, K., Ross, V., Hawgood, J., Spence, S. H., & De Leo, D. (2017). The impact of a student's suicide: Teachers' perspectives. *Journal of Affective Disorders, 207*, 276–281. https://doi.org/10.1016/j.jad.2016.09.058

Kovac, S. H., & Range, L. M. (2000). Writing projects: Lessening undergraduates' unique suicidal bereavement. *Suicide & Life-Threatening Behavior, 30*(1), 50–60. https://doi.org/10.1111/j.1943-278X.2000.tb01064.x

Krysinska, K., & Andriessen, K. (2017). Online suicide bereavement and support. In K. Andriessen, K. Krysinska, & O. T. Grad (Eds.), *Postvention in action: The international handbook of suicide bereavement support* (pp. 197–211). Hogrefe.

Krysinska, K., Currier, D., & Andriessen, K. (2024). Evaluation of a new online program for children bereaved by suicide: The views of children, parents, and facilitators. *Archives of Suicide Research: Official Journal of the International Academy for Suicide Research, 28*(1), 384–398. https://doi.org/10.1080/13811118.2023.2185559

Leaune, E., Ravella, N., Vieux, M., Poulet, E., Chauliac, N., & Terra, J. L. (2019). Encountering patient suicide during psychiatric training: An integrative, systematic review. *Harvard Review of Psychiatry, 27*(3), 141–149. https://doi.org/10.1097/HRP.0000000000000208

Leaune, E., Cuvillier, B., Vieux, M., Pacaut-Troncin, M., Chalancon, B., Perez, A. F., Haesebaert, J., Chauliac, N., Poulet, E., & Durif-Bruckert, C. (2020). The SUPPORT-S protocol study: A postvention program for professionals after patient or user suicide. *Frontiers in Psychology, 11*, 805. https://doi.org/10.3389/fpsyg.2020.00805

Leaune, E., Rouzé, H., Lestienne, L., Bislimi, K., Chalancon, B., Morgiève, M., Grandgenèvre, P., Vaiva, G., Laplace, N., Poulet, E., & Haesebaert, J. (2022). The needs, use and expectations of people bereaved by suicide regarding online resources: An online survey. *International Journal of Environmental Research and Public Health, 19*(19), 12156. https://doi.org/10.3390/ijerph191912156

Lestienne, L., Leaune, E., Haesebaert, J., Poulet, E., & Andriessen, K. (2021). An integrative systematic review of online resources and interventions for people bereaved by suicide. *Preventive Medicine, 152*(Pt 1), 106583. https://doi.org/10.1016/j.ypmed.2021.106583

Lezine, D. (2016). Suicide prevention through personal experience. In R. C. O'Connor & J. Pirkis (Eds.), *The international handbook of suicide prevention* (2nd ed.). Wiley. https://doi.org/10.1002/9781118903223.ch38

Linde, K., Treml, J., Steinig, J., Nagl, M., & Kersting, A. (2017). Grief interventions for people bereaved by suicide: A systematic review. *PLoS One, 12*(6), e0179496. https://doi.org/10.1371/journal.pone.0179496

Lyra, R. L., McKenzie, S. K., Every-Palmer, S., & Jenkin, G. (2021). Occupational exposure to suicide: A review of research on the experiences of mental health professionals and first responders. *PLoS One, 16*(4), e0251038. https://doi.org/10.1371/journal.pone.0251038

Maple, M., Pearce, T., Sanford, R., Cerel, J., Castelli Dransart, D. A., & Andriessen, K. (2018). A systematic mapping of suicide bereavement and postvention research and a proposed strategic research agenda. *Crisis, 39*(4), 275–282. https://doi.org/10.1027/0227-5910/a000498

Maples, M. F., Packman, J., Abney, P., Daugherty, R. F., Casey, J. A., & Pirtle, L. (2005). Suicide by teenagers in middle school: A postvention team approach. *Journal of Counseling & Development, 83*(4), 397–405. https://doi.org/10.1002/j.1556-6678.2005.tb00361.x

Marshall, D., Moutier, C., Rosenblum, L., Miara, C., & Posner, M. (2018). *After a suicide: A toolkit for schools*. American Foundation for Suicide Prevention, Suicide Prevention Resource Center, & Education Development Center. https://sprc.org/wp-content/uploads/2022/12/AfteraSuicideToolkitforSchools-3.pdf

McDaid, C., Trowman, R., Golder, S., Hawton, K., & Sowden, A. (2008). Interventions for people bereaved through suicide: Systematic review. *The British Journal of Psychiatry: the Journal of Mental Science, 193*(6), 438–443. https://doi.org/10.1192/bjp.bp.107.040824

McDonnell, S., Nelson, P. A., Leonard, S., McGale, B., Chew-Graham, C. A., Kapur, N., Shaw, J., Smith, S., & Cordingley, L. (2020). Evaluation of the impact of the PABBS suicide bereavement training on clinicians' knowledge and skills. *Crisis, 41*(5), 351–358. https://doi.org/10.1027/0227-5910/a000646

McDonnell, S., Flynn, S., Shaw, J., Smith, S., McGale, B., & Hunt, I. M. (2022). Suicide bereavement in the UK: Descriptive findings from a national survey. *Suicide & Life-Threatening Behavior, 52*(5), 887–897. https://doi.org/10.1111/sltb.12874

Mitchell, A. M., & Terhorst, L. (2017). PTSD symptoms in survivors bereaved by the suicide of a significant other. *Journal of the American Psychiatric Nurses Association, 23*(1), 61–65. https://doi.org/10.1177/1078390316673716

Mitchell, A. M., Kim, Y., Prigerson, H. G., & Mortimer-Stephens, M. (2004). Complicated grief in survivors of suicide. *Crisis, 25*(1), 12–18. https://doi.org/10.1027/0227-5910.25.1.12

National Action Alliance for Suicide Prevention. (2014). *Suicide attempt survivors task force*. The Action Alliance. https://theactionalliance.org/events/suicide-attempt-survivors-task-force

Neimeyer, R. A. (2000). Searching for the meaning of meaning: grief therapy and the process of reconstruction. *Death Studies, 24*(6), 541–558. https://doi.org/10.1080/07481180050121480

Nelson, P. A., Cordingley, L., Kapur, N., Chew-Graham, C. A., Shaw, J., Smith, S., McGale, B., & McDonnell, S. (2020). 'We're the First Port of Call' – Perspectives of Ambulance Staff on responding to deaths by suicide: A qualitative study. *Frontiers in Psychology, 11*, 722. https://doi.org/10.3389/fpsyg.2020.00722

Pfeffer, C. R., Jiang, H., Kakuma, T., Hwang, J., & Metsch, M. (2002). Group intervention for children bereaved by the suicide of a relative. *Journal of the American Academy of Child and Adolescent Psychiatry, 41*(5), 505–513. https://doi.org/10.1097/00004583-200205000-00007

Pirkis, J., Bantjes, J., Dandona, R., Knipe, D., Pitman, A., Robinson, J., Silverman, M., & Hawton, K. (2024). Addressing key risk factors for suicide at a societal level. *The Lancet. Public Health, 9*(10), e816–e824. https://doi.org/10.1016/S2468-2667(24)00158-0

Pitman, A., Osborn, D., King, M., & Erlangsen, A. (2014). Effects of suicide bereavement on mental health and suicide risk. *The Lancet. Psychiatry, 1*(1), 86–94. https://doi.org/10.1016/S2215-0366(14)70224-X

Pitman, A. L., Osborn, D. P., Rantell, K., & King, M. B. (2016). Bereavement by suicide as a risk factor for suicide attempt: A cross-sectional national UK-wide study of 3432 young bereaved adults. *BMJ Open, 6*(1), e009948. https://doi.org/10.1136/bmjopen-2015-009948

Pitman, A., McDonald, K., Logeswaran, Y., Lewis, G., Cerel, J., Lewis, G., & Erlangsen, A. (2024). The role of depression and use of alcohol and other drugs after partner suicide in the association between suicide bereavement and suicide: Cohort study in the Danish population. *Psychological Medicine, 54*(9), 2273–2282. https://doi.org/10.1017/S0033291724000448

Poijula, S., Dyregrov, A., Wahlberg, K. E., & Jokelainen, J. (2001). Reactions to adolescent suicide and crisis intervention in three secondary schools. *International Journal of Emergency Mental Health, 3*(2), 97–106.

Ross, V., Kõlves, K., & De Leo, D. (2021). Exploring the support needs of people bereaved by suicide: A qualitative study. *Omega, 82*(4), 632–645. https://doi.org/10.1177/0030222819825775

Schlichthorst, M., Ozols, I., Reifels, L., & Morgan, A. (2020). Lived experience peer support programs for suicide prevention: A systematic scoping review. *International Journal of Mental Health Systems, 14*, 65. https://doi.org/10.1186/s13033-020-00396-1

Scocco, P., Zerbinati, L., Preti, A., Ferrari, A., & Totaro, S. (2019). Mindfulness-based weekend retreats for people bereaved by suicide (Panta Rhei): A pilot feasibility study. *Psychology and Psychotherapy, 92*(1), 39–56. https://doi.org/10.1111/papt.12175

Séguin, M., Bordeleau, V., Drouin, M. S., Castelli-Dransart, D. A., & Giasson, F. (2014). Professionals' reactions following a patient's suicide: Review and future investigation. *Archives of Suicide Research: Official Journal of the International Academy for Suicide Research, 18*(4), 340–362. https://doi.org/10.1080/13811118.2013.833151

Séguin, M., Roy, F., & Boilar, T. (2019). *Programme de postvention: être prêt à agir à la suite d'un suicide*. Association québécoise de prévention du suicide (AQPS).

Shear, K., & Shair, H. (2005). Attachment, loss, and complicated grief. *Developmental Psychobiology, 47*(3), 253–267. https://doi.org/10.1002/dev.20091

Shear, K., Frank, E., Houck, P. R., & Reynolds, C. F. (2005). Treatment of complicated grief: A randomized controlled trial. *JAMA, 293*(21), 2601–2608. https://doi.org/10.1001/jama.293.21.2601

Solomon, P. (2004). Peer support/peer provided services underlying processes, benefits, and critical ingredients. *Psychiatric Rehabilitation Journal, 27*(4), 392–401. https://doi.org/10.2975/27.2004.392.401

Stroebe, M., & Schut, H. (1999). The dual process model of coping with bereavement: Rationale and description. *Death Studies, 23*(3), 197–224. https://doi.org/10.1080/074811899201046

Supiano, K. P. (2012). Sense-making in suicide survivorship: A qualitative study of the effect of grief support group participation. *Journal of Loss and Trauma, 17*(6), 489–507. https://doi.org/10.1080/15325024.2012.665298

Supiano, K. P., Haynes, L. B., & Pond, V. (2017). The transformation of the meaning of death in complicated grief group therapy for survivors of suicide: A treatment process analysis using the meaning of loss codebook. *Death Studies, 41*(9), 553–561. https://doi.org/10.1080/07481187.2017.1320339

Szumilas, M., & Kutcher, S. (2011). Post-suicide intervention programs: A systematic review. *Canadian journal of public health = Revue canadienne de sante publique, 102*(1), 18–29. https://doi.org/10.1007/BF03404872

Takahashi, C., Chida, F., Nakamura, H., Akasaka, H., Yagi, J., Koeda, A., Takusari, E., Otsuka, K., & Sakai, A. (2011). The impact of inpatient suicide on psychiatric nurses and their need for support. *BMC Psychiatry, 11*, 38. https://doi.org/10.1186/1471-244X-11-38

Tamworth, M., Killaspy, H., Billings, J., & Gibbons, R. (2022). Psychiatrists' experience of a peer support group for reflecting on patient suicide and homicide: A qualitative study. *International Journal of Environmental Research and Public Health, 19*(21), 14507. https://doi.org/10.3390/ijerph192114507

Testoni, I., Francescon, E., De Leo, D., Santini, A., & Zamperini, A. (2019). Forgiveness and blame among suicide survivors: A qualitative analysis on reports of 4-year self-help-group meetings. *Community Mental Health Journal, 55*(2), 360–368. https://doi.org/10.1007/s10597-018-0291-3

Tur, C., Campos, D., Suso-Ribera, C., Kazlauskas, E., Castilla, D., Zaragoza, I., García-Palacios, A., & Quero, S. (2022). An Internet-delivered Cognitive-Behavioral Therapy (iCBT) for Prolonged Grief Disorder (PGD) in adults: A multiple-baseline single-case experimental design study. *Internet Interventions, 29*, 100558. https://doi.org/10.1016/j.invent.2022.100558

Visser, V. S., Comans, T. A., & Scuffham, P. A. (2014). Evaluation of the effectiveness of a community-based crisis intervention program for people bereaved by suicide. *Journal of Community Psychology, 42*(1), 19–28. https://doi.org/10.1002/jcop.21586

Wainwright, V., Cordingley, L., Chew-Graham, C. A., Kapur, N., Shaw, J., Smith, S., McGale, B., & McDonnell, S. (2020). Experiences of support from primary care and perceived needs of parents bereaved by suicide: A qualitative study. *The British Journal of General Practice: The Journal of the Royal College of General Practitioners, 70*(691), e102–e110. https://doi.org/10.3399/bjgp20X707849

Watling, D., Preece, M., Hawgood, J., Bloomfield, S., & Kõlves, K. (2022). Developing an intervention for suicide prevention: A rapid review of lived experience involvement. *Archives of Suicide Research: Official Journal of the International Academy for Suicide Research, 26*(2), 465–480. https://doi.org/10.1080/13811118.2020.1833799

Wittouck, C., Van Autreve, S., Portzky, G., & van Heeringen, K. (2014). A CBT-based psychoeducational intervention for suicide survivors: A cluster randomized controlled study. *Crisis, 35*(3), 193–201. https://doi.org/10.1027/0227-5910/a000252

World Health Organization, & International Association for Suicide Prevention. (2008). *Preventing suicide: How to start a survivors' group*. World Health Organization.

World Health Organization. (2021). *LIVE LIFE: An implementation guide for suicide prevention in countries*. World Health Organization.

Zisook, S., Shear, M. K., Reynolds, C. F., Simon, N. M., Mauro, C., Skritskaya, N. A., Lebowitz, B., Wang, Y., Tal, I., Glorioso, D., Wetherell, J. L., Iglewicz, A., Robinaugh, D., & Qiu, X. (2018). Treatment of complicated grief in survivors of suicide loss: A HEAL report. *The Journal of Clinical Psychiatry, 79*(2), 17m11592. https://doi.org/10.4088/JCP.17m11592

Chapter 11
The Impact of Suicide on Clinical Teams: Exploring the Needs of Mental Health Professionals

Susana Morales-Silva

11.1 The Impact of Suicide on Clinical Teams

The occurrence of suicide not only results in an irreparable loss but also profoundly affects families, loved ones, and the broader environment. This impact extends to the clinical teams involved in the patient's care, including psychiatrists, psychologists, psychotherapists, social workers, nurses, general practitioners, counselors, and other medical support staff (Foley & Kelly, 2007).

Given the prevalence of suicide, it is a challenge that clinicians across all health subspecialties are likely to encounter at some point in their careers. Research indicates that 22–39% of psychologists and 51–82% of psychiatrists will experience at least one patient suicide during their professional lives (Lafayette & Stern, 2004). Moreover, approximately 10% of healthcare professionals are at increased risk of suicide themselves following the death of a patient under their care (Dransart et al., 2015).

A patient's suicide can have profound emotional and professional impacts on healthcare professionals, often resulting in significant and enduring emotional reactions like intense grief (Foley & Kelly, 2007). It is recognized as an occupational hazard that can profoundly affect clinicians' personal and professional lives (Sandford et al., 2021). Emotionally, it may trigger a range of responses, including shock, sadness, anger, frustration, self-reproach, self-doubt, social withdrawal, decreased self-esteem, disrupted relationships, symptoms of posttraumatic stress disorder, anxiety, depression, and lowered self-confidence (Foley & Kelly, 2007). Professionally, it may lead to heightened caution in suicide risk assessments, defensiveness in patient interactions, and even thoughts of early retirement. These events

S. Morales-Silva (✉)
Red de Salud UC-Christus, Pontificia Universidad Católica de Chile, Santiago, Chile

Millennium Institute for Research in Depression and Personality (MIDAP), Santiago, Chile

Á. Jiménez-Molina, V. Martínez (eds.), *New Perspectives on Suicidal Behavior*, Depression and Personality, https://doi.org/10.1007/978-3-031-96037-6_11

can cause clinicians to question their skills and develop fears related to their practice (Courtenay & Stephens, 2001). Unfortunately, many professionals face these challenges without adequate institutional support, often relying on informal emotional support from colleagues and peer groups (Dewar et al., 2000). This peer support plays a crucial role in postvention, a coordinated response designed to mitigate the negative impacts of such traumatic events and promote healing and recovery among those affected (Sandford et al., 2021). The literature underscores the importance of training, postvention support, and preparation to mitigate such incidents' distress and long-term effects. Effective management strategies are essential to address these risks and protect against staff burnout, ultimately enhancing professional practices (Foley & Kelly, 2007).

This chapter reviews the literature on the impact of patient suicide on mental health practitioners. It explores the emotional and professional challenges faced by therapists whose patients died by suicide during therapy. Through an inquiry into the perspectives of three therapists (Morales, 2023), the chapter examines their initial reactions and the evolution of their views over time, highlighting the profound emotional toll and the critical need for institutional and personal support. It also delves into the immediate and long-term effects on their clinical practice, showing how these experiences have shaped their professional perspectives. The chapter concludes by identifying key clinical concerns and offering recommendations to improve support for mental health professionals.

This chapter explores the experiences of three psychotherapists who faced the suicide of a patient during ongoing therapy. These therapists, differing in gender, age, theoretical orientation, and years of experience, were interviewed to understand their reactions and perspectives on the event. The interviews were analyzed in detail using content analysis to uncover explicit and underlying themes (White & Marsh, 2006). The analysis revealed key insights into the therapists' emotional reactions, the impact on their clinical practice, the understanding they developed over time, the emotional support they received, and the long-term effects on their professional and personal lives. Recommendations are made for institutions and therapists to support professionals in similar situations better. The thematic script used in the interviews is included in Table 11.1.

11.2 Emotional Reactions After Learning the News of the Patient's Suicide

The existing literature consistently reports a range of emotional responses among healthcare professionals after learning of a patient's suicide, including guilt, blame, shock, anger, sadness, anxiety, self-doubt, poor concentration, disturbed sleep, decreased appetite, apathy, preoccupation with work, and grief (Linke et al., 2002; Sandford et al., 2021).

Table 11.1 Thematic script used in the interviews

Experiences of the interviewees:
1. About what happened: Circumstances (triggering event, childhood trauma antecedent), alliance (bonding agreement, tasks, and objectives), and time the psychotherapy began
2. Impact this had on their own experience (emotional)
3. Impact this had on how they conducted other psychotherapeutic processes (in terms of technique)
4. Whether they had any support during this crisis period, from whom, and in what form
5. Whether there was any institutional intervention (in case the psychotherapeutic process took place under the wing of an institution)
6. Topics that they considered relevant aspects after the past event
7. Recommendation to therapists to prepare for and mitigate the impact of this experience
8. Some recommendations that they made to institutions to prepare professionals and mitigate the impact of this experience

Source: Author's creation based on the literature

Dransart et al. (2015) highlight that the emotional and traumatic reactions experienced by professionals following a patient's suicide often stem from a strong connection to the patient, which intensifies their response. There is also evidence of increased suicidal behaviors or ideation among practitioners after such events (Castelli Dransart et al., 2014). Dransart et al. (2015) categorize practitioners' reactions based on their characteristics and the support they receive, revealing varying impacts across different groups. Professionals in low-impact groups who experienced less emotional distress and fewer adverse reactions in their clinical practice had received significant institutional and peer support, anticipated the patient's death, and felt less emotionally connected to the patient. These practitioners typically had more theoretical and clinical training, particularly in suicide risk assessment, and their relationships with the patients were brief and had ended before the patient's death (Dransart et al., 2014, 2015).

In contrast, higher-impact groups included professionals who felt emotionally close to and responsible for the patient, maintained contact until the patient's death, and had longer relationships with the patient. These professionals perceived the support they received as inadequate and had encountered more patient suicides but received less training compared to their colleagues. As a result, they were more likely to experience significant emotional and professional repercussions, including leaving the practice or avoiding patients at risk of suicide altogether (Dransart et al., 2015). The study underscores the importance of support and training in mitigating these risk factors. Those in low-impact groups benefited from more comprehensive training and adequate support, while the most impacted individuals received comparatively less training and support (Dransart et al., 2015).

The experience of a patient's suicide can elevate the risk of suicidal thoughts or attempts among healthcare practitioners, as noted by Kleespies et al. (1993). Similar emotions were observed among therapists in our inquiry, who reported intense feelings of devastation and self-doubt immediately after learning of their patient's death. One therapist described the experience as "devastating" (EIII.P10), while another felt "inept" (EII.P14). These intense emotional reactions often significantly change how professionals interact with patients, affecting their self-confidence and approach to clinical practice.

11.3 Effects of Suicide on Clinical Practice

Research indicates that the suicide of a patient can have significant consequences for clinical practice, particularly among psychiatry trainees, with 68% reporting such impacts (Courtenay & Stephens, 2001). Similar effects have been observed in psychologists, including increased focus on detecting signs of suicidal ideation, more conservative record-keeping, and greater reliance on peer consultation (Trimble et al., 2000). Additionally, practitioners may exhibit avoidance behaviors, such as reluctance to accept high-risk patients, heightened attention to legal aspects, and a desire to change jobs, along with a tendency to distance themselves emotionally and physically from patients (Cryan et al., 1995; Linke et al., 2002).

Further studies reveal that clinicians often respond by engaging in more detailed record-keeping, adopting more conservative attitudes toward terminating treatment, and being more vigilant about patients' thoughts of suicide (Finlayson & Graetz Simmonds, 2018; Halligan & Corcoran, 2021). In a study involving nurses, Wang et al. (2016) found that poor training in suicide risk and prejudgments, such as avoiding discussions about death, contributed to increased fear, guilt, stress, and excessive vigilance among staff. These factors and a lack of training may lead to emotional regulation patterns such as venting to family and friends and avoiding critical patients.

Moreover, clinicians may struggle with professional uncertainty and self-doubt, affecting their confidence in decision-making (Finlayson & Graetz Simmonds, 2018). They might also seek guidance from colleagues more frequently, prioritize swift hospitalization and posttreatment monitoring, and become more willing to consider suicide as a potential outcome (Menninger, 1991; Sandford et al., 2021).

The interviewed therapists reported that learning of a patient's suicide had a profound impact on their clinical work. Some reacted impulsively by discontinuing treatment with high-risk patients, while others became overly cautious in their practice. As one therapist expressed, "I referred all the patients at risk of suicide … I did not dare" (EII.P16). These experiences often led to significant emotional and professional challenges, resulting in noticeable shifts in how they interacted with patients and approached their clinical practice.

11.4 The Understanding of Suicide Over Time

The unexpected nature of a patient's suicide often leads to an immense shock, deeply affecting healthcare staff. This sense of shock reverberates through all aspects of their work, and the emotional and practical impacts can persist for years. Research shows that these effects, such as heightened vigilance, increased focus on risk assessment, stricter adherence to policies, and containment methods such as enhanced observation and improved environmental security, can continue for up to 10 years (Bowers et al., 2006). These strategies, while intended to prevent future suicides, have shown mixed effectiveness.

Moreover, the long-term emotional impacts of such events remain significant, influencing clinical practice even years later (Bowers et al., 2006; Sanders et al., 2005). Over time, some emotions, such as guilt and recrimination, gradually diminish as professionals come to terms with the realization that they did their best and that not all suicides can be prevented (Ting et al., 2006). However, disbelief is the only emotion reported to decrease significantly over time (Saini et al., 2016). Despite this gradual emotional reconciliation, the profound impact of a patient's suicide continues to shape clinicians' approaches to care in the long term.

Over time, the interviewees experienced a shift in their understanding of their patients' suicides, leading to a reduction in self-recriminations and feelings of guilt about their clinical actions. This process allowed them to recognize both the help they provided and what more they could have done while still questioning themselves to some extent: "It has helped me to think that (my intervention prolonged her life), but I still question myself" (EII.P22). The literature and interviewees' experiences highlight a significant shift in perspective as time passes. This gradual understanding reflects the dynamic nature of human cognition, showcasing the potential for growth and greater insight over time.

11.5 Emotional Support Received by Practitioners

Observations by psychotherapists regarding the aftermath of a patient's suicide highlight the varying degrees of psychological support described in different studies. A recurring theme is the high value placed on individual emotional support, whether informal or through confidential supervision, especially when institutional support is lacking (Tillman, 2006). When formal support was available, personal debriefing sessions and group supervision specifically designed for processing the effects of a patient's suicide were particularly appreciated. In contrast, clinical team meetings or informational sessions were less valued during the crisis (Gibbons et al., 2019).

Support from colleagues and family members also played a crucial role in helping clinicians cope with the distress. The nature of this support greatly influenced the recovery process—understanding responses were found to be reparative, while hostile responses made recovery more difficult (Castelli Dransart et al., 2014). Additionally, meeting with the deceased patient's family, although emotionally demanding, could provide psychological relief (Tillman, 2006).

Interviewed therapists echoed these findings, recalling the significant support they received from peers and family. One therapist noted, "The supervisor and coworkers were an enormous support to help me rebuild" (EII.P15), while another emphasized, "From my spouse … I felt welcomed and supported" (EIII.P38, 39). Both the literature and therapists' experiences underline the importance of emotional support following a patient's suicide, often occurring informally and in the absence of institutional support. This highlights the need for healthcare institutions to formalize emotional readiness programs for prevention and postvention efforts.

11.6 Endured Emotionality Over the Years

The emotional impact of a patient's suicide on practitioners typically has both immediate and long-lasting effects. While the reviewed literature often explores the short- and medium-term impacts on clinical teams, it generally does not delve deeply into the emotional effects that persist over the years (Gulfi et al., 2016). When examining long-term effects, studies primarily focus on variables related to the extent of the impact on practitioners and the types of support that help mitigate negative consequences. These factors are commonly categorized into five overarching themes.

1. Practitioner characteristics, among which stand out a greater number of years in practice, had a protective influence on impact (Draper et al., 2014).
2. Patient characteristics, where the younger age of the patient who dies by suicide was shown to have a more significant impact (Wurst et al., 2013).
3. The therapeutic relationship includes the strength of the relationship (Bowers et al., 2006), emotional closeness (Castelli Dransart et al., 2014), disliking the patient (Dewar et al., 2000), and difficulty with emotional contact with the patient (Davidsen, 2011; Pieters et al., 2003). These factors are reported as increasing the negative impact of the patient's death.
4. Responses from others were fear of reactions from relatives and being blamed for them, which were associated with higher levels of suffering (Gibbons et al., 2019).
5. Concerns regarding litigation and exposure were moderate, and extreme distress was presented with the prospect of litigation and media exposure (Murphy et al., 2022).

Health service–level interventions are recommended to reduce professional distress and its impact on practice over time (Foley & Kelly, 2007). Despite some emotional relief over the years, interviewees reported that lingering doubts and unresolved feelings about the events persist, as one noted, "What happened is still not very clear to me" (EII.P1). Both the literature and the interviewees underscore the importance of support and containment from the health service, particularly valuing informal support, which plays a crucial role in helping practitioners emotionally cope with the aftermath of a patient's suicide.

11.7 A Deeper Understanding of What Occurred at That Time

The emotional impact of losing a patient to suicide often prompts clinicians to develop a new understanding of the event over time (Bowers et al., 2006). Studies indicate that such experiences deeply affect clinicians' emotional state and professional practice, influencing their relationship with themselves as practitioners and with their patients (Ting et al., 2006). This heightened awareness can lead to better recognition of the limitations in preventing suicide, fostering a more realistic acceptance of suicide as a potential outcome in treatment (Gulfi et al., 2016; Kleespies et al., 1993; Linke et al., 2002; Ting et al., 2006). Over time, this awareness may help reduce self-doubt and gradually restore confidence in their professional abilities (Saini et al., 2016). An important factor in understanding these events is recognizing that severe depression in patients can negatively affect the therapeutic alliance, contributing to the eventual outcome (Richardson-Vejlgaard et al., 2013).

The narratives of the three interviewed psychotherapists reveal the experience of an unexpected relational breakdown, which had a profound emotional and professional impact. This led to self-recrimination, revision of interventions, and lingering questions about what could have been done differently. These intense emotions—guilt, blame, shock, anger, sadness, anxiety, and grief—can persist for a long time, though self-recrimination may diminish as new explanations and understandings emerge (Corbella & Botella, 2003).

The intense emotional impact of a patient's suicide often leaves therapists with lingering guilt and uncertainty, even after they recover from the initial shock and come to a relative understanding of the event. This experience creates a sense of relational rupture, where the therapeutic alliance and bond with the patient failed to withstand the suicide crisis (Corbella & Botella, 2003). Therapists often reflect on the disconnect between their understanding of the therapeutic relationship and the patient's internal experience, which they can only infer from the patient's ultimate act of withdrawal from life. As one therapist noted, "He was clear from the point of view of alliance, bond, and objectives, but he fulfilled it partially because he did not bring up everything that worried him internally" (EIII.P25).

The literature and preliminary findings suggest that, despite extensive clinical training and expertise, therapists continue to face significant technical and emotional challenges when working with patients at risk of suicide. This underscores the need to incorporate specialized assessment and intervention methodologies that address clinical needs and enhance therapists' ability to regulate their emotions and manage feelings of powerlessness in such challenging situations.

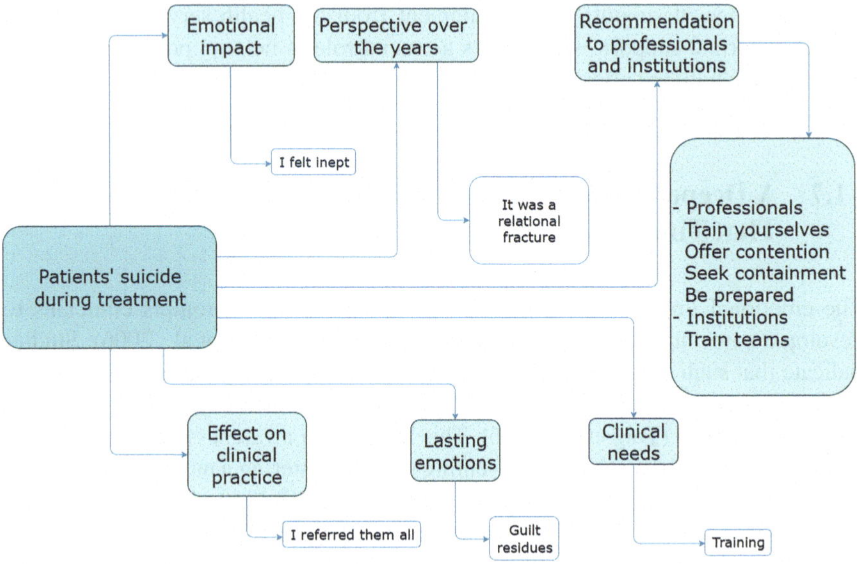

Fig. 11.1 Psychotherapists' perspectives on patients who die by suicide during treatment

A graphic representation of what three psychotherapists reported about the loss of a patient who died by suicide during treatment is summarized in Fig. 11.1.

11.8 Recommendations for Therapists and Institutions

The reviewed studies emphasize the significant challenges faced by clinical teams, particularly psychotherapists when dealing with the suicide of active patients. They strongly recommend additional measures to prepare professionals for the possibility of losing a patient to suicide and to establish effective emotional support systems for healthcare teams (Bowers et al., 2006). The research also highlights the traumatic impact of patient suicide on practitioners, noting that current professional training does not adequately prepare them for such an event. This gap is particularly concerning for mental health professionals, and the studies advocate for incorporating this topic into career training, starting at the undergraduate level. This training should include assessments, interventions, and postvention strategies, particularly for mental health teams (Sandford et al., 2021). Furthermore, the studies underscore the benefits of informal peer support in helping clinicians process the emotional aftermath of a patient's suicide. They suggest structured support mechanisms within institutions to assist clinical teams during crises (Courtenay & Stephens, 2001).

In postvention, researchers emphasize the importance of institutional preparedness and a comprehensive response to patient suicides, given their recurring nature.

A key recommendation is to adopt a non-blame-seeking approach that fosters a learning culture through thorough event reviews, thereby reducing the traumatic impact on clinicians (Sandford et al., 2021). Therapists have stressed the necessity of integrating suicide risk assessment and intervention training into the basic curriculum for psychotherapists, viewing it as a minimum requirement for handling patients at risk: "Training needs to be part of the basic training of psychotherapists" (EI.P52, P54).

The literature review and study findings indicate that professional training should encompass both the assessment and treatment of individuals at risk of suicide, as well as postvention support for clinicians. Such support should be facilitated by healthcare institutions through both formal and informal mechanisms. Clinical teams frequently face considerable psychological challenges in processing the suicide of a patient, whether inpatient or outpatient. This distress may give rise to blame-shifting, feelings of professional inadequacy, and disruptions within the workplace. The impact is often compounded by fragile support structures and a lack of trust among colleagues, who may be hesitant to acknowledge perceived personal failures. In this context, it is crucial to convene the staff involved during the immediate postvention period—ideally in a dedicated session rather than at the end of a routine clinical meeting—to collectively remember the deceased and reconstruct the sequence of events. Such settings offer a psychologically safe space for clinicians to express emotions such as sadness, anger, and helplessness, and to share their reflections. Importantly, they also provide an opportunity to draw shared lessons from the experience, framing the death as a result of systemic shortcomings, rather than attributing blame to individual practitioners.

11.9 Addressing the Emotional and Professional Impact of Patient Suicide

The experience of a patient's suicide can be devastating for clinicians, with impacts like bereavement that may persist for years. This underscores the need for better preparation and support for mental health professionals, particularly psychotherapists, who may encounter such events during their practice.

Informal emotional support from health services plays a crucial role. However, there is also a pressing need for comprehensive training in evaluating and treating at-risk patients and postvention strategies supported by health institutions. Recognizing emotionality as an inherent part of psychotherapy, understanding the limits of what therapists can control, and clearly defining therapist–patient responsibilities are essential. Emphasizing teamwork and self-care is vital to preventing burnout and ensuring that professionals are equipped to handle the emotional challenges of their work.

Given the challenges of working with patients at risk of suicide, we need a team-based approach rather than working in isolation. This work is emotionally demanding and interdisciplinary, requiring significant responsibility. Therapists must prioritize self-care to avoid overinvolvement, recognize their emotional responses, and maintain clear boundaries. In the therapeutic setting, it is crucial to balance technical expertise with human compassion, encouraging emotional expression and validating the patient's suffering without endorsing the idea of dying.

It is also important to consider psychosocial factors contributing to suicide risk, advocating for a multidisciplinary team approach that allows for shared responsibilities and a comprehensive assessment of the patient's complexities and vulnerabilities (de la Parra et al., 2022, 2023). Ultimately, clinical teams must recognize that patient suicide is an inherent risk in the profession and that the decision to die by suicide is ultimately an internal one made by the patient, beyond the direct control of healthcare professionals (Rothes et al., 2013).

The World Health Organization (WHO, 2022) emphasizes the critical importance of both prevention and postvention in addressing suicide risk. This is particularly relevant for psychotherapists and mental health professionals, who may themselves be at increased risk of suicidal ideation and attempts after losing a patient to suicide (Kleespies et al., 1993). Recognizing that suicide risk affects a broad spectrum of society, the WHO advocates for primary prevention as a communal responsibility.

Primary prevention in mental health involves actively engaging in practices that promote self-care and reduce vulnerability to suicide. Shneidman (1993) highlighted the importance of addressing "psychache"—intense psychological pain—as a key factor in suicide prevention, suggesting that without psychache, the risk of suicide diminishes. To support these goals, the following strategies are recommended:

- Engagement in self-care: Encourage individuals to adopt self-care practices that enhance physical, mental, and emotional well-being. This includes mindfulness, relaxation techniques, regular exercise, and sufficient sleep.
- Mitigating vulnerability to suicide: Focus on proactive actions that address personality and social vulnerabilities, thereby reducing the risk of suicidal ideation or self-harm.
- Improving intra- and interpersonal skills: Develop skills for managing emotions and relationships effectively. This includes improving communication, coping mechanisms, problem-solving, and conflict resolution, all of which can serve as protective factors against suicide.
- Promoting healthy lifestyle habits: Encourage healthy lifestyle choices, such as maintaining a balanced diet, staying physically active, avoiding substance abuse, and engaging in fulfilling activities, which are essential for overall well-being and mental health.

These strategies aim to foster resilience and reduce suicide risk across the community, with further details provided in Table 11.2.

Building on the literature review and initial research into the impact of patient suicide on psychotherapists, future studies should focus on how institutional and professional peer support mechanisms can be structured to offer formalized care in

Table 11.2 Prevention strategies in mental health

Developing intrapersonal skills
Accepting feeling unpleasant emotions
Practicing exercises for calming intrusive thoughts and letting them go
Recognizing one's value, even in one's differences
Being able to identify and express emotions
Being able to focus on what is necessary in the moment
Sustaining a kind and respectful relationship with oneself
Developing interpersonal skills
Recognizing the value of others, even in others' differences
Incorporating assertive communication strategies
Promoting conflict resolution skills
Developing a kind and respectful relationship with others
Promoting healthy lifestyle habits
Maintaining some level of physical activity
Keeping stress as low as possible (limited work schedules)

Note: Based on WHO recommendations (World Health Organization, 2022)

these situations. Enhancing training for professionals who work closely with at-risk populations is particularly crucial. By examining the implementation of robust support systems within institutions and peer networks, researchers can better address the needs of those affected by patient suicide. This proactive approach is vital for fostering resilience and safeguarding the well-being of mental health professionals who frequently face such complex challenges.

Acknowledgments I extend my gratitude to the UC-Christus Health Network, the Millennium Institute for Research in Depression and Personality (MIDAP), and the Department of Psychiatry at Pontificia Universidad Católica de Chile. I also want to thank the UC-MIDAP team members who have collaborated with me in research and clinical practice related to suicide prevention since 2007.

References

Bowers, L., Simpson, A., Eyres, S., Nijman, H., Hall, C., Grange, A., & Phillips, L. (2006). Serious untoward incidents and their aftermath in acute inpatient psychiatry: The Tompkins Acute Ward Study. *International Journal of Mental Health Nursing, 15*(4), 226–234. https://doi.org/10.1111/j.1447-0349.2006.00428.x

Castelli Dransart, D. A., Gutjahr, E., Gulfi, A., Kaufmann Didisheim, N., & Séguin, M. (2014). Patient suicide in institutions: Emotional responses and traumatic impact on Swiss Mental Health Professionals. *Death Studies, 38*(5), 315–321. https://doi.org/10.1080/07481187.2013.766651

Corbella, S., & Botella, L. (2003). La alianza terapeutica: Historia, investigacion y evaluacion/Therapeutic alliance: History, research and assessment. *Anales de Psicologia, 19*(2), 205–221.

Courtenay, K. P., & Stephens, J. P. (2001). The experiencie of patient suicida among trainees in psychiatry. *Psychiatric Bulletin, 51*, 51–52. https://doi.org/10.1016/s0140-6736(02)88363-5

Cryan, E. M. J., Kelly, P., & McCaffrey, B. (1995). The experience of patient suicide among Irish psychiatrists. *Psychiatric Bulletin, 19*(1), 4–7. https://doi.org/10.1192/pb.19.1.4

Davidsen, A. S. (2011). And then one day hed shot himself. Then I was really shocked: General practitionersreaction to patient suicide. *Patient Education and Counseling, 85*(1), 113118. https://doi.org/10.1016/j.pec.2010.08.020

de la Parra, G., Crempien, C., Morales, S., Zúñiga, A. K., & Errázuriz, A. (Eds.). (2023). *Herramientas psicoterapéuticas para elmanejo de pacientes con depresión: Una guía para el trabajo en atención primaria (APS)*. Ediciones UC.

de la Parra, G., Zúñiga, A. K., Crempien, C., Morales, S., Errázuriz, A., Martínez, P., Aravena, C., & Ferrari, T. (2022). Delphi validation of a psychotherapeutic competencies training protocol for the treatment of depression in PHC. *Studies in Psychology*, 17–36. https://doi.org/10.1080/02109395.2022.2127239

Dewar, I., Eagles, J., Klein, S., Gray, N., & Alexander, D. (2000). Psychiatric trainees' experiences of, and reactions to, patient suicide. *Psychiatric Bulletin, 24*(1), 20–23. https://doi.org/10.1192/pb.24.1.20

Dransart, D. A. C., Heeb, J. L., Gulfi, A., & Gutjahr, E. M. (2015). Stress reactions after a patient suicide and their relations to the profile of mental health professionals. *BMC Psychiatry, 15*(1), 1–9. https://doi.org/10.1186/s12888-015-0655-y

Draper, B., Kõlves, K., De Leo, D., & Snowdon, J. (2014). The impact of patient suicide and sudden death on health care professionals. *General Hospital Psychiatry, 36*(6), 721–725. https://doi.org/10.1016/j.genhosppsych.2014.09.011

Finlayson, M., & Graetz Simmonds, J. (2018). Impact of client suicide on psychologists in Australia. *Australian Psychologist, 53*(1), 23–32. https://doi.org/10.1111/ap.12240

Foley, S. R., & Kelly, B. D. (2007). When a patient dies by suicide: Incidence, implications and coping strategies. *Advances in Psychiatric Treatment, 3*(2), 134–138. https://doi.org/10.1192/apt.bp.106.002501

Gibbons, R., Brand, F., Carbonnier, A., Croft, A., Lascelles, K., Wolfart, G., & Hawton, K. (2019). Effects of patient suicide on psychiatrists: Survey of experiences and support required. *BJPsych Bulletin, 43*(5), 236–241. https://doi.org/10.1192/bjb.2019.26

Gulfi, A., Castelli Dransart, D. A., Heeb, J. L., & Gutjahr, E. (2016). The impact of patient suicide on the professional practice of Swiss psychiatrists and psychologists. *Academic Psychiatry, 40*(1), 13–22. https://doi.org/10.1007/s40596-014-0267-8

Halligan, P., & Corcoran, P. (2021). The impact of patient suicide on the psychiatrist. *Australasian Psychiatry, 29*(6), 705–706. https://doi.org/10.1177/10398562211003603

Kleespies, P. M., Penk, W. E., & Forsyth, J. P. (1993). The stress of patient suicidal behavior during clinical training: Incidence, impact, and recovery. *Professional Psychology: Research and Practice, 24*(3), 293–303. https://doi.org/10.1037/0735-7028.24.3.293

Lafayette, J. M., & Stern, T. A. (2004). The impact of a patient's suicide on psychiatric trainees: A case study and review of the literature. *Harvard Review of Psychiatry, 12*(1), 49–55. https://doi.org/10.1080/10673220490279152

Linke, S., Wojciak, J., & Day, S. (2002). The impact of suicide on community mental health teams: Findings and recommendations. *Psychiatric Bulletin, 26*(2), 50–52. https://doi.org/10.1192/pb.26.2.50

Menninger, W. (1991). Patient suicide and its impact on the psychotherapist. *Bulletin of the Menninger Clinic, 55*(2), 216–227.

Morales, S. (2023). *Indagación exploratoria de la vivencia del terapeuta ante el suicidio de un paciente con proceso en curso*. Informe de estudio. Santiago: MIDAP.

Murphy, P. T., Clogher, L., Van Laar, A., O'Regan, R., McManus, S., McIntyre, A., O'Connell, A., Geraghty, M., Henry, G., & Hallahan, B. (2022). The impact of service user's suicide on mental health professionals. *Irish Journal of Psychological Medicine, 39*(1), 74–84. https://doi.org/10.1017/ipm.2019.4

Pieters, G., De Gucht, V., Joos, G., & De Heyn, E. (2003). Frequency and impact of patient suicide on psychiatric trainees. *European Psychiatry, 18*(7), 345349. https://doi.org/10.1016/j.eurpsy.2003.02.003

Richardson-Vejlgaard, R., Broudy, C., Brodsky, B., Fertuck, E., & Stanley, B. (2013). Predictors of psychotherapy alliance in Borderline Personality Disorder. *Psychotherapy Research, 23*(5), 539–546. https://doi.org/10.1080/10503307.2013.801001

Rothes, I. A., Scheerder, G., Van Audenhove, C., & Henriques, M. R. (2013). Patient suicide: The experience of flemish psychiatrists. *Suicide and Life-threatening Behavior, 43*(4), 379–394. https://doi.org/10.1111/sltb.12024

Saini, P., Chantler, K., While, D., & Kapur, N. (2016). Do GPs want or need formal support following a patient suicide?: A mixed methods study. *Family Practice, 33*(4), 414–420. https://doi.org/10.1093/fampra/cmw040

Sandford, D. M., Kirtley, O. J., Thwaites, R., & O'Connor, R. C. (2021). The impact on mental health practitioners of the death of a patient by suicide: A systematic review. *Clinical Psychology and Psychotherapy, 28*(2). https://doi.org/10.1002/cpp.2515

Sanders, S., Jacobson, J., & Ting, L. (2005). Reactions of mental health social workers following a client suicide completion: A qualitative investigation. Omega: *Journal of Death and Dying, 51*(3), 197–216. https://doi.org/10.2190/D3KH-EBX6-Y70P-TUGN

Shneidman, E. S. (1993). Commentary: Suicide as psychache. *Journal of Nervous and Mental Disease, 181*(3), 145–147. https://doi.org/10.1097/00005053-199303000-00001

Tillman, J. G. (2006). When a patient commits suicide: An empirical study of psychoanalytic clinicians. *International Journal of Psychoanalysis, 87*(1), 159–177. https://doi.org/10.1516/417a-ucdf-3u7q-0en6

Ting, L., Sanders, S., & Power, R. (2006). Reactions after a Client Suicide. *Social Work, 51*, 329–342.

Trimble, L., Jackson, K., & Harvey, D. (2000). Client suicidal behaviour: Impact, interventions, and implications for psychologists. *Australian Psychologist, 35*(3), 227–232. https://doi.org/10.1080/00050060008257483

Wang, S., Ding, X., Hu, D., Zhang, K., & Huang, D. (2016). A qualitative study on nurses' reactions to inpatient suicide in a general hospital. *International Journal of Nursing Sciences, 3*(4), 354–361. https://doi.org/10.1016/j.ijnss.2016.07.007

White, M. D., & Marsh, E. E. (2006). Content analysis: A flexible methodology. *Library Trends, 55*(1), 22–45. https://doi.org/10.1353/lib.2006.0053

World Health Organization. (2022). *WHO Guidelines on mental health at work*. https://www.who.int/publications/i/item/9789240053052, https://www.who.int/publications/i/item/9789240057944

Wurst, F. M., Kunz, I., Skipper, G., Wolfersdorf, M., Beine, K. H., Vogel, R., et al. (2013). How therapists react to patient's suicide: Findings and consequences for health care rofessionals' wellbeing. *General Hospital Psychiatry, 35*(5), 565–570. https://doi.org/10.1016/j.genhosppsych.2013.05.00

Index

Á. Jiménez-Molina, V. Martínez (eds.), *New Perspectives on Suicidal Behavior, Depression and Personality*, https://doi.org/10.1007/978-3-031-96037-6

The manufacturer's authorised representative in the EU is Springer Nature Customer Service Centre GmbH, Europaplatz 3, 69115 Heidelberg, Germany. If you have any concerns regarding our products, please contact ProductSafety@springernature.com

Printed and bound by CPI Group (UK) Ltd, Croydon, CR0 4YY
30/09/2026
02225588-0001